MICROBIOLOGY IN PATIENT CARE

Second Edition

H. I. WINNER
M.A., M.D., F.R.C.P., F.R.C.Path.,
Professor of Medical Microbiology
Charing Cross Hospital Medical School, University of London
Consultant Bacteriologist, Charing Cross Group of Hospitals

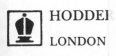 HODDER

LONDON

D1335302

ISBN 0 340 22969 1 Boards
ISBN 0 340 22970 5 Paperback

First printed 1969. Reprinted 1970 (with revisions), 1972 (twice),
1973, 1974, 1975 (with revisions)
Second Edition 1978. Reprinted 1979 (twice)

Printed and bound in Great Britain
for Hodder and Stoughton Educational
a division of Hodder and Stoughton Ltd,
Mill Road, Dunton Green, Sevenoaks, Kent
by Biddles Ltd, Guildford, Surrey

EDITORS' FOREWORD

The scope of this series has increased since it was first established, and it now serves a wide range of medical, nursing and ancillary professions, in line with the present trend towards the belief that all who care for patients in a clinical context have an increasing amount in common.

The texts are carefully prepared and organised so that they may be readily kept up to date as the rapid developments of medical science demand. The series already includes many popular books on various aspects of medical and nursing care, and reflects the increased emphasis on community care.

The increasing specialisation in the medical profession is fully appreciated and the books are often written by Physicians or Surgeons in conjunction with specialist nurses. For this reason, they will not only cover the syllabus of training of the General Nursing Council, but will be designed to meet the needs of those undertaking training controlled by the Joint Board of Clinical Studies set up in 1970.

To Nina, Jonathan, Linda, Simon, Daniel, and Rachel

PREFACE TO SECOND EDITION

My aim in this book has been to give nurses and other people who work in hospitals a sound guide which will help them in their everyday work. The subject of Microbiology looms large in the management of patients in a modern hospital, in the use of modern instruments, apparatus and surgical materials, and in the general deportment of hospital staff.

On the other hand, no one wants a book burdened with jargon, and I have tried to keep technical terms down to the minimum.

I have received valuable help and advice from Dr. H. J. Andrews, Dr. A. Beck, Dr. J. C. Coleman, Mr. Eric Crozier, Dr. A. Gerken, Miss Valerie Hunt, S.R.N., Miss Helga Legge, Mr. T. Ridgewell, and Dr. D. J. M. Wright. The public Trustee and the Society of Authors kindly gave permission for the inclusion of a passage from *The Doctor's Dilemma* by Bernard Shaw. To all these I am grateful.

Finally I must thank my publishers for their encouragement, forbearance and assistance.

H. I. WINNER
Charing Cross Hospital Medical School
London

CONTENTS

CHAPTER 1

INTRODUCTION

Early history

It has been known for thousands of years that some diseases could be conveyed from one person to another; in other words, that they were **infectious.** In the Bible and other ancient writings occur descriptions of contagious diseases, which are those spread by direct contact, and of measures taken to prevent infection. Leprosy, bubonic plague and smallpox can all be recognised in antique literature, though diagnosis was vague, and similar diseases were often confused with one another.

Attacks of infectious disease were usually attributed to divine wrath, which could manifest itself either on the individual or on the community. Nothing at all was known about microbes, and their existence in any scientific sense was not suspected. None the less, in certain parts of the world there grew up a rule-of-thumb knowledge, based on trial and error, of how to prevent and to deal with infection.

Perhaps the most remarkable example of this was the practice of variolation, or inoculation with smallpox. This was practised in China and other countries apparently for hundreds of years before the invention of vaccination by Jenner in 1798. Another example is the widespread use of mould preparations for the treatment of superficial wounds, which foreshadowed the discovery of antibiotics.

Early scientists and alchemists believed in the doctrine of spontaneous generation, and considered that living organisms could come into existence from non-living dirt.

The discovery of bacteria

The science of Bacteriology can be said to have started in the seventeenth century, with the discovery of bacteria by **Leeuwenhoek** of Delft. It was not until two hundred years later, in the nineteenth century, that microbes were found to be the cause of disease. Perhaps the greatest of the early bacteriologists was the French chemist **Louis Pasteur** (1822-1895). He discovered many pathogenic microbes, and also invented means of culturing them in the laboratory. He showed that it was possible to weaken or 'attenuate' dangerous bacteria, and to use these for immunising. Pasteur also showed the fallacies of the theories of spontaneous generation, the doctrine that living things could arise out of non-living matter. He demonstrated that this did not take place, and that bacteria only flourished where bacteria had existed before.

The list of Pasteur's discoveries is a very long one; there are few men to whom humanity owes more. The remarkable thing is that he added greatly to medical knowledge although he was not a qualified doctor of medicine. He was a chemist, and he had to overcome much prejudice from medical men.

The German physician **Robert Koch** (1843-1910) was another whose interest in bacteria led him to many fundamental discoveries. Perhaps his most important discovery was that of the tubercle bacillus and of the mechanism whereby it causes disease.

Vaccination

Empirical knowledge of the facts of bacteriology and immunity came long before the discovery of pathogenic microbes. Thus, at the end of the eighteenth century, half a century before the work of Pasteur and Koch, **Edward Jenner** introduced the practice of vaccination. This followed his observation that an attack of cowpox, a trivial disease in man, could confer immunity to the fatal disease smallpox. However, Jenner knew nothing about the microbes concerned, and it was not for over a hundred years that the smallpox virus was discovered.

Sepsis, antisepsis, and asepsis

The care of the sick in hospitals, up to the middle of the nineteenth century, reflected the general ignorance about the dangers of microbial infection. Especially was this true of surgery. There was no conception of asepsis, of antisepsis, or of cross-infection. No attempts were made to keep surgical wounds clean, either at operation or afterwards. Consequently, most surgical wounds became infected, and post-operative fatalities were commonplace. Patients who did not die after operation from the results of sepsis often suffered serious and prolonged illness. This is not surprising when one considers that surgeons often operated in their ordinary everyday clothes, without gowns or masks, and that nurses and others in the operating theatres also wore ordinary clothes. Many surgeons did not even wash their hands before operations. Surgery at this time was necessarily crude by present-day standards. It was largely confined to traumatic surgery, the treatment of civil and wartime injuries and the drainage of abscesses, with some specific internal procedures such as 'cutting for the stone', and the removal of superficial tumours. There was virtually no 'internal surgery', abdominal surgery or laparotomies, and no chest or brain surgery other than the treatment of accidents or wounds. Obstetrics was extremely crude and septic, and thousands of mothers every year died of puerperal fever, infection contracted in childbirth. **Semmelweis**, who worked in Vienna in the middle of the nineteenth century, showed that puerperal sepsis was due to infection of the mothers from the hands of obstetricians and midwives. He succeeded in reducing the incidence of sepsis by persuading operators and their assistants to disinfect their hands. However, he met with much opposition, and his work was neglected for a time.

It was left to an English surgeon, **Joseph Lister**, to apply to surgery the recently discovered facts and theories about sepsis propounded by Semmelweis and Pasteur.

Lister, who was at the time Professor of Surgery at Glasgow, was deeply concerned about the large number of his patients who contracted serious sepsis after being operated upon. He sought a method of preventing this. He was much struck by the work of Pasteur on fermentation, and he conceived the idea that the putrefaction of surgical wounds was a process similar to the fermentation of sugars by microbes. He introduced the **antiseptic** principle into surgery, whereby chemical antiseptics were liberally used during operations to kill any contaminating microbes.

It was a logical step from antisepsis to **asepsis**, the exclusion of microbes by the techniques practised today in operating theatres throughout the world.

The application of antiseptic principles to surgery opened the way for great advances of surgical technique, and this advance was hastened by the development of asepsis. Today it is possible to operate with a high degree of safety from infection on any part of the body. Without aseptic techniques, this would not have been possible, and abdominal surgery, thoracic surgery and brain surgery could never have developed.

The development of modern nursing

The application of medical knowledge and techniques would itself have been much frustrated if there had not been corresponding advances in the principles of looking after the sick in hospitals. These advances were led by an Englishwoman, **Florence Nightingale**, who was one of the greatest figures in medicine in the nineteenth century. At this time, nursing was not a highly respected profession. Miss Nightingale's first contribution, when she was still a young woman, was to organise a completely new type of hospital in which the nursing was performed by well-educated women with a high sense of vocation. They were capable of learning and applying the basic scientific concepts, such as those of bacteriology, on which modern hospital practice is founded.

The story of how the British Government enlisted Florence Nightingale's help in reorganising hospitals for the troops during the Crimean War is well known. After the Crimean War, Florence Nightingale returned to England and became the leading authority in all aspects of nursing care and hospital administration. Her book *Notes on Nursing* is the classic text on the subject and is still worth serious study. She advised on the planning and organisation of hospitals in India as well as in England, and wrote standard textbooks on the subject. The principles laid down by Miss Nightingale on such matters as the correct spacing of beds in hospitals are still of value in planning in such a way as to reduce the spread of infection. But perhaps her main contribution was to create the modern concept of the hospital nurse, and to lay down clear principles for the training of nurses.

Viruses

Most of the bacteria which cause disease were discovered in the last fifty years of the last century. At the beginning of this century the existence of still smaller microbes, the viruses, was suspected, and the first viruses were discovered. It was soon realised that viruses cause at least as much illness as bacteria, and that virus diseases, from mild infections such as the common cold to serious ones like smallpox, were widespread throughout the world.

At present we are still in the middle of the stage of discovery. Every year, several new viruses are isolated. New vaccines for dealing with virus infections are constantly being devised, and there is an intense search in progress for antibiotics active against viruses. Perhaps it can now be said that the greater part of the work of discovery is done, and that the chief problem now is to apply the knowledge gained in recent years.

Public Health

The discovery of specific microbes brought about a great change in public health. At last it was possible to put the practice of drainage and sanitation on to a scientific basis, so that cities, towns, and the country are healthier and safer places to live in than they have ever been in the past.

Immunology

There followed the development of immunology — using injections of microbes or of extracts of microbes deliberately to induce immunity. The first successful large scale applications of this were the use by Professor **Almroth Wright**, during the Boer War, of killed vaccines against typhoid, which greatly reduced the mortality due to this cause. Since that time, many other vaccines have been introduced, bringing great reductions in the incidence of many diseases such as diphtheria, tuberculosis, poliomyelitis and tetanus. Today, no sooner is a new microbe isolated than intensive attempts are made to prepare vaccines to immunise people against it. Within the last few years, this has happened in the case of poliomyelitis, and it is happening now in the case of measles, rubella (german measles) and cold viruses.

In recent years, interest in immunology has greatly increased. One reason is the development of sero-diagnostic tests for a wide variety of suspected infections. Another is the development of transplant surgery, in which the immunological reactions of the recipient are of great importance. Substances such as 'transfer factor' have been discovered in serum.

Antibiotics

Another period of great advance in medicine was introduced by the discovery of penicillin by **Alexander Fleming** in 1928, though it was over ten years before this was successfully applied to the treatment of human infections. This era of antibiotics marks as big a step forward as any that has been made in the past. As a result, most of the bacterial infections which twenty years ago used to be fatal, or which often caused long and crippling illness, have now been rendered comparatively trivial. Pneumococcal and streptococcal infections are examples of infection which have become much less dangerous. Moreover, every bacterial infection may now be treated by one of the many available antibiotics, though the success of this treatment varies. In some infections it is almost always successful; in others its value is doubtful. Infections by large viruses, such as that of typhus, can also be treated by antibiotics, and there are good prospects of antibiotics effective against other virus infections.

The result of all these advances is that serious infections are no longer the most important causes of death in many countries. Human beings live longer, and they live lives more free from infection, than at any time in the past.

CHAPTER 2

CHARACTERISTICS OF
DISEASE-PRODUCING MICROBES

Microbes which cause diseases are all small objects which cannot be seen except by the use of microscopes. They cover a wide range of sizes. The largest are about 1/100 of 1mm (10 micrometres) in length. The smallest are about one thousandth of this size. The comparative sizes of some of these are shown in Figure 1.

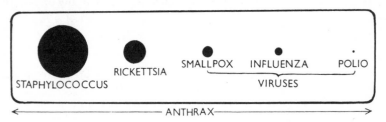

Fig. 1. Comparative sizes of some microbes.
The length of the anthrax bacillus is approximately 1/100 of 1mm or 10 micrometres

The largest microbes illustrated are about the same size as cells of the human body, such as the red blood cells. The smallest ones, however, are little bigger than large molecules of protein.

The larger microbes are the bacteria, the smaller ones are the viruses. The differences between them are not only those of size. Most bacteria can be cultured or grown under artificial conditions in media which are not alive, such as bottles of broth or culture plates. Viruses, however, can only be grown inside the living cells of animals or tissue cultures. While some of the largest viruses resemble small bacteria, the smallest viruses are much less complicated and resemble molecules of nucleoprotein which have the power to reproduce themselves; there is much doubt as to whether they should be regarded as 'alive' at all.

The rickettsias are a group of microbes whose size and general properties are similar to those of the largest viruses. In this book, for the sake of simplicity, they are included with viruses.

In addition to bacteria and viruses, there are minute fungi and protozoa which case disease. These are mostly larger than the largest bacteria, but are still too small to be seen with the naked eye and are about the same order of size as the cells of the human body.

Microbes which cause disease are said to be pathogenic. These are only a small proportion of the total number of microbes. Some non-pathogenic bacteria, such as the nitrogen-fixing bacteria of the soil, play an important part in agriculture. Others are responsible for important industrial processes such as the production of cheese from milk. Many species of pathogenic bacteria infect animals other than man, including cold-blooded animals such as fishes, and invertebrates. Similarly, there are viruses and microscopic fungi which infect other animals and plants, and there are also viruses, the bacteriophages, which infect bacteria.

In this book we are concerned only with microbes that infect human beings.

The Morphology of Bacteria

The most important types of bacteria are the following:

1. **Cocci** (Berries). These are spherical or nearly so. They may have the shape of soccer balls, rugger balls, kidneys or spearheads.

Fig. 2. Types of cocci: staphylococci, streptococci, pneumococci, neisserias

Staphylococci grow in culture as clusters looking like bunches of grapes.
Streptococci form chains, which may be short or long.
Neisserias, sometimes called diplococci, appear as pairs of kidney-shaped microbes facing towards one another.
Pneumococci also appear in pairs, as spearheads.

2. **Bacilli** (Rods). These may be regular and rectangular, or irregular and beaded; they may be relatively long and thin, or short and fat. They may have flagella, in which case they are motile. Examples are the **colon bacillus** (*Escherichia coli*), the **anthrax bacillus**, the **diphtheria bacillus**, and the **'vibrio'** of cholera, which is curved and has a flagellum.

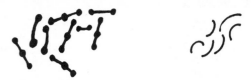

Fig. 3. Diphtheria bacilli, vibrios

3. **Spirochaetes**. These are long slender organisms which are spirally coiled and motile. Examples are the **treponema** of syphilis and the **leptospira** of Weil's disease.

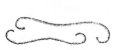

Fig. 4. Treponema, leptospira

4. **Actinomycetes**. These are short rod-like forms which may join together to become long branching filaments.

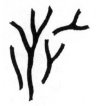

Fig. 5. Actinomycetes

The Structure and Morphology of Viruses

Viruses multiply only in living cells, and the particles usually studied in the laboratory are inert resting phases of their life-cycle. These particles vary greatly in size and shape. There are filamentous forms, round forms, some of which are very irregular, and tadpole-like forms.

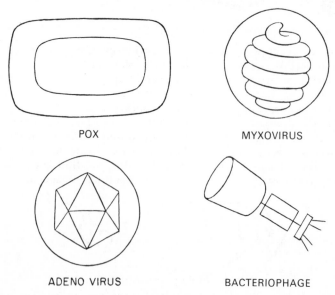

POX   MYXOVIRUS

ADENO VIRUS   BACTERIOPHAGE

Fig. 6. The shapes of some viruses

    The largest viruses resemble the smallest bacteria in many ways, and are sensitive, like bacteria, to tetracycline and certain other antibiotics. The smallest viruses, however, have a much simpler structure. They consist of little more than a few molecules of nucleoprotein, which is the fundamental substance that makes up living matter. There are two varieties of nucleic acid, **deoxyribonucleic acid**, or **DNA**, and **ribonucleic acid**, or **RNA**. Viruses contain one or other of these.

    Some of the smaller viruses, such as the poliomyelitis virus and various plant viruses, have been prepared in crystalline form.

The Morphology of Pathogenic Fungi

Pathogenic fungi, like all other fungi, consist largely of rounded bodies called **spores** and filamentous threads called **hyphae**, which are matted together to form a **mycelium**. Often the spores are contained in **sporangia** of various shapes as shown.

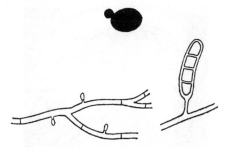

Fig. 7. Some pathogenic fungi

Culture and Multiplication of Microbes

Food left exposed to the atmosphere 'goes bad'. This means that bacteria and fungi from the surrounding air settle and grow on it. In the laboratory, special bacterial foods called **media** are prepared to grow these organisms. Some media are jellies, made of a seaweed product called **agar**, to which various nutritive substances such as blood and glucose may be added. Round plastic or glass dishes called **petri dishes** are used to hold the media. Sometimes fluid media are used; these are filtered soups or broths, kept in test-tubes or screw-topped bottles. Some bacteria grow in the presence of oxygen and are called **aerobic**. Others will not grow in the presence of oxygen and are called **anaerobic**. These have to be grown in special jars in an artificial atmosphere of hydrogen and nitrogen (see Fig. 9). Some will grow in either aerobic or anaerobic atmospheres; these are called **facultative anaerobes**.

In the laboratory a large number of different media are used to grow bacteria, and there is much skill in devising suitable **selective** media, which will encourage the growth of the particular bacteria in which one is interested but not others.

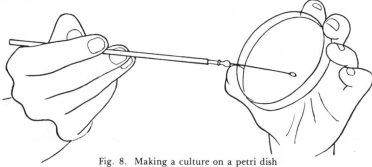

Fig. 8. Making a culture on a petri dish

With two exceptions, all bacteria known to be pathogenic can be cultured artificially in this way. These exceptions are two of the most important types of disease-producing bacteria, the leprosy bacillus and treponema which carries syphilis and other diseases. These have never been cultured artificially on non-living media.

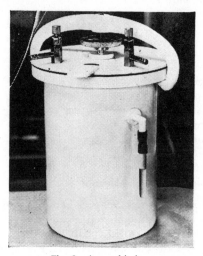

Fig. 9. Anaerobic jar

The Multiplication of Bacteria

Bacteria reproduce themselves by cell division; the method differs with different types of bacteria (see Fig. 10).

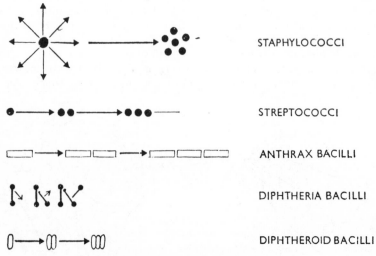

Fig. 10. Methods of multiplication of some bacteria

Under the most favourable conditions in the laboratory, bacteria can double their numbers in about twenty minutes. This rate of growth cannot be maintained indefinitely, however; it depends on a readily available food supply, the removal of waste products, and adequate ventilation.

Moreover, this optimal rate is not achieved until the bacteria have become accustomed to their environment. After subculture, the growth of bacteria goes through a well defined cycle, which is illustrated in Figure 11.

At first, the number of organisms does not change very much; this is the period of adaptation to their new environment and is known as the **lag phase**. Then occurs the period of intense growth at maximum speed; this is the **logarithmic phase**. As the available food supply declines, the rate of growth decreases, and increasing numbers of microbes die, so that the total number remains fairly stable; this is the **stationary phase**. Finally, as the food supply becomes exhausted and the concentration of waste products becomes toxic, the numbers diminish; this is the **phase of decline**.

It is possible to maintain the logarithmic rate of growth indefinitely by continually replenishing the food supply and removing waste products, and by providing a continuous supply of oxygen. This is the **continuous culture** method used in the commercial manufacture of antibiotics.

In the human body, an infecting microbe goes through phases of growth analogous to those illustrated, modified however by the reaction of the human host to infection. After pathogenic microbes enter a host, there is a **latent phase** during which the microbes become accustomed to their new

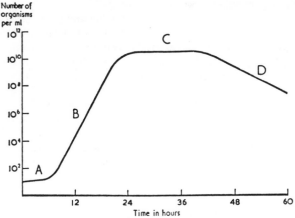

Fig. 11. The growth cycle of bacteria, showing how the numbers of living organisms in a culture changes as time goes on

A: lag phase   C: stationary phase
B: logarithmic phase   D: phase of decline

environment. They then start to multiply, and this corresponds to the logarithmic phase observed in the laboratory. If the infection is overwhelming, the logarithmic phase may continue until the patient dies.

More often, however, the body defences of the host cause the rate of multiplication to slow down and eventually to stop completely.

Spores

When conditions are unfavourable for them to multiply in the way described above, some types of bacteria are capable of developing into resistant forms or **spores**, in which they may remain in a state of suspended animation until conditions become favourable again, when they become

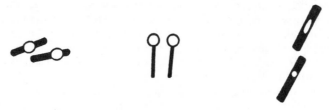

Fig. 12. Spores:
A: Clostridium welchii; B: Clostridium tetani; C: Anthrax bacillus

converted into the ordinary **vegetative** forms. The chief spore-bearing bacteria include some of the most dangerous pathogens, notably the bacteria of **gas gangrene, tetanus** and **anthrax**.

Spores are difficult to kill. They may resist boiling for several hours. They can survive cold and drying and the action of chemical disinfectants in much higher concentrations that would kill vegetative bacteria. When dry, spores are blown about freely in the air. It is obvious, therefore, that they may be extremely dangerous carriers of infection. It is in order to kill spore-bearing organisms that drastic methods of disinfection have to be used in hospitals, such as steam under pressure in the autoclave, hot-air ovens, and infra-red assembly lines. These methods are discussed in Chapter 9.

The gas gangrene and tetanus bacilli are **anaerobic**, that is to say, the spores germinate and the bacteria reproduce only in the absence of oxygen.

The Identification of Bacteria in the Laboratory

The first step towards identifying bacteria in the laboratory is to culture them. This is usually done on solid media in petri dishes.

The swab or loop containing infected material is wiped over the plate in the manner shown, so as to thin out the inoculum of living bacteria. This plate is then incubated at 37° C, the temperature of the human body, which is the best temperature for the growth of pathogenic bacteria. Each

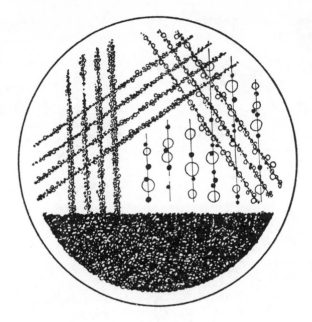

Fig. 13. Showing the pattern of inoculating a plate. The circles represent colonies of bacteria which have grown during incubation

single bacterium deposited on the plate starts to grow and multiply according to the process already described. In a few hours, each microbe has become millions of microbes, and has formed a visible circular **colony** of bacteria.

Colonies of different types of bacteria have different appearances, and these can often be distinguished easily by naked eye examination.

On suitable media, some bacteria produce characteristic effects which enable them to be identified. Thus, **haemolytic streptococci** contain a toxin which destroys red blood cells. Colonies of these organisms on blood agar are therefore surrounded by a halo of colourless medium, in which the blood cells have been destroyed. The appearance of these haemolytic colonies is characteristic.

Coliform bacilli are grown on media, such as MacConkey's medium, which contain bile salts. These salts suppress the growth of most other types of bacteria. Usually, lactose and an indicator dye is incorporated in the medium; this enables one to tell at a glance, after incubation, whether or not the organism has fermented the lactose and produced acid from it.

Diphtheria bacilli grow well on plates of blood agar containing potassium tellurite, on which they produce black colonies with characteristic shapes and surface textures, different from those of other bacteria.

From the colonies on plates, smears of the microbes can be made on microscope slides and these can be stained and examined (see Fig. 14).

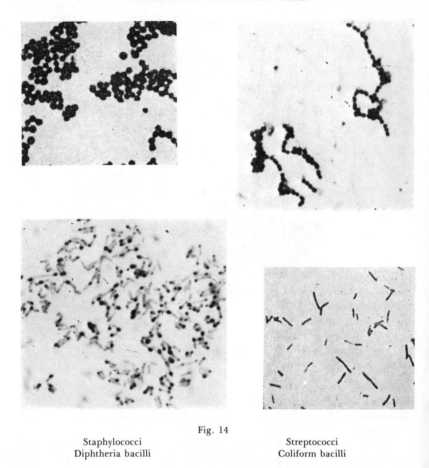

Fig. 14

Staphylococci   Streptococci
Diphtheria bacilli   Coliform bacilli

Staining Methods

The staining methods employed make use of the fact that different chemical substances within the body of the bacteria are stained different colours by different stains. The commonest method is **Gram's method**. In this method, the magnesium ribonucleate which is present in some bacteria is stained a deep purple with a mixture of violet dye and iodine, and this purple stain cannot readily be washed out by alcohol. Bacteria which stain in this way by Gram's method are called **gram positive**. When other bacteria without magnesium ribonucleate are stained by Gram's method, the purple dye can easily be washed out by alcohol. These microbes are called **gram negative**. This differentiation into gram-positive and gram-negative organisms is an important method of differentiating bacteria. A list of some gram-positive and gram-negative bacteria is given in the table:

SOME GRAM-POSITIVE AND GRAM-NEGATIVE BACTERIA

Gram-positive	*Gram-negative*
Staphylococci	Escherichia coli (Coliform bacillus)
Streptococci	Proteus
Diphtheria bacillus (Corynebacterium diphtheriae)	Pseudomonas aeruginosa
	Typhoid bacillus (Salmonella typhi)
Gas gangrene bacillus (Clostridium welchii)	Paratyphoid bacilli (Salmonella paratyphi A, B and C)
Tetanus bacillus (Clostridium tetani)	Food poisoning bacilli (other salmonellas)
Anthrax bacillus	Dysentery bacilli (Shigellas)
Tubercle bacillus (Mycobacterium tuberculosis)	Gonococcus (Neisseria gonorrhoeae)
Lactobacillus	Meningococcus (Neisseria meningitidis)
	Plague bacillus (Yersinia pestis)
	Haemophilus influenzae
	Brucella
	Whooping cough bacillus (Bordetella pertussis)
	Spirochaetes

The method used for staining the tubercle bacillus depends on the fact that the waxy envelope of this organism is difficult to penetrate with stain, and hot strong stain has to be used. Once stained, the organism holds the stain well and cannot be decolourised with strong acid and alcohol. This bacillus is therefore said to be 'acid-fast', and the staining method is named after its inventors the **Ziehl-Neelsen** or 'Z.N.' method.

When suspected tuberculous material, such as sputum, is stained, concentrated hot red dye is applied, and then the slide is washed with concentrated sulphuric acid and alcohol. After this treatment the tubercle bacilli, if they are present, remain red, but all the rest of the slide is colourless. The slide is then counterstained with a blue or a yellow dye. When examined under the microscope, tubercle bacilli can readily be seen as they stand out red against a blue or yellow background.

Another staining method is used for the identification of the diphtheria bacillus, which stains the granules a different colour from the rest of the organism. This double colour staining is called metachromatic staining.

Other Tests for Identifying Bacteria

It may be necessary to confirm the identity of the bacteria by special tests. For example the organisms of the coli-typhoid-dysentery group, which live in the bowel, are all gram-negative bacilli which look alike under the microscope. One of the ways they differ is in the sugars they ferment. When solutions of particular sugars, such as glucose, lactose, sucrose, and so on, are placed in the bottles of culture medium in which one of these bacilli are growing, the microbe will ferment some of the sugars but not others. Different organisms of the group may be differentiated by seeing which of a number of sugars they will ferment, and whether or not they produce gas during the fermentation process. Thus, *E. coli* ferments lactose, but the salmonella and dysentery organisms do not (with minor exceptions). If a lactose-fermentation test is done on an organism, the result indicates whether or not the organism is likely to be a salmonella or dysentery bacillus, and therefore a dangerous type of bowel infection, or a comparatively harmless *E. coli*.

Serological tests are also much used. These employ antisera against various bacteria, which may have some easily seen effect on the specific bacteria, such as agglutinating or clumping them; some types of bacteria can be identified by seeing which antisera agglutinate them. This is the way in which coliform, enteric and dysentery bacilli are finally identified. In identifying viruses, a more complicated serological test called the **complement fixation test** may be used.

Another type of identification technique makes use of fluorescent dyes. These are chemically linked to bacterial antisera, and smears of the microbe being identified are treated with the fluorescent-stained antisera. The specific antiserum will then cause its particular bacteria to fluoresce in ultra-violet light, and this fluorescence can be seen under the microscope. Other antisera will not have this effect. This fluorescent-staining technique offers a relatively simple and quick method of identifying certain types of bacteria.

How Bacteria cause Disease—Toxins

Bacteria mostly cause disease by virtue of poisonous substances or **toxins** which they produce. In some cases, the poisons diffuse away from the bacteria into the body of the patient. These are called **exotoxins**, and examples are those of the diphtheria bacillus and the tetanus bacillus. The bacilli can remain at a particular place in the host and produce disease a long way away.

Some toxins are extremely powerful. Thus the botulinus toxin, produced by *Clostridium botulinum*, is the most poisonous substance known, and about 1/100mg will kill a human being.

Many bacteria produce numerous exotoxins, which are individually not very strong but which together damage the host considerably and enable the bacterium to multiply and spread within the host tissues. Thus, among the toxins produced by pathogenic staphylococci are those which damage the red cells, the white cells, and the tissue cells. There are also toxins which coagulate plasma and which reduce surface tension, thus enabling other toxins to spread in the tissues. Another staphylococcal toxin, the enterotoxin, acts on the small intestine producing symptoms of food poisoning. Pathogenic streptococci produce a powerful haemolysin, or toxin, which destroys the red blood cells, in addition to toxins which act on the other cells of the body and on the skin. The gas gangrene bacillus is another microbe which produces numerous varied exotoxins.

In other bacteria, the toxins are part of the actual bacterial cell, and are called **endotoxins**. The bacterium only causes disease if it is in direct contact with the tissues of the host. An example is the **typhoid** bacillus.

The Multiplication of Viruses

Viruses and rickettsias can only multiply inside suitable living cells such as those of an animal, a chick embryo in its egg, or a tissue culture. These are all used in the laboratory for the culture of viruses.

The first step towards virus multiplication is the invasion by the virus of a cell in which it can multiply. The virus particle then breaks down into its constituent molecules of nucleic acid within the cell. The virus as a single entity disappears: it 'dissolves' in the cell. The next step is the utilisation by the virus subunits of the metabolic enzymes of the host cell, which it takes over, causing the enzymes to use the cell substance to manufacture more virus units instead of doing their normal job of keeping the cell going.

When the supply of nutrients inside the host cell is exhausted, the virus molecules reform themselves into virus particles, the cell ruptures, and the numerous particles leave it to invade more cells.

Thus a single virus enters the cell, and after the process of multiplication, many viruses leave the cell.

In the process described above, the host cell is destroyed by the virus. This happens in most virus diseases. However, there is some evidence that in certain infections the cycle may not complete itself with the destruction of the host cell, but the virus may remain 'latent' inside the cell, in equilibrium with it and not destroying it. Many people believe that the latent infection of cells by viruses in this way may be one of the causes of malignant change in cells.

The Resistance of Microbes

Most bacteria are killed by a temperature well below that of boiling water — between 60° and 80° C (60° is the lowest temperature at which, for most people, a glass of water feels unbearably hot to the back of the hand). Some but not many are killed by cooling to refrigerator temperature. On the other hand many **spores** (see page 12) survive being boiled for several hours and can also survive drying, refrigeration, and lack of food supply.

Viruses are all killed by temperatures of 60°-80° C. On the other hand, they are extremely resistant to cold. Very low temperatures, well below that of the ordinary refrigerator or deep freeze cabinet, are used to preserve them alive.

The subject of resistance to heat, and disinfection in general, is dealt with in Chapter 9.

CHAPTER 3

THE SPREAD OF MICROBES
AND THE PATHS OF INFECTION

The natural habitat of most disease-producing microbes is other human being or animals. When microbes infect humans, they have usually come either directly or indirectly from these sources. Microbes which are found in the air get there from the secretions, or from the mouth and throat, of humans or animals. Microbes in the soil get there by being dropped in the faeces of animals.

A person is said to be **'infected'** with a particular microbe when he harbours it in such a state that it can maintain itself by multiplying. The infected person is called the **host**. A host can be infected without being ill; infection does not necessarily mean disease, and many infected hosts are healthy **carriers** — that is, they may transmit the microbes to other people and hence may be a source of infection, without themselves becoming ill. These 'carriers' are discussed further below.

Normal Flora of Humans

Every healthy person is infected with a variety of microbes, which are said to be **commensal** — meaning that they live on the host but do not do him any harm. In fact their presence may do positive good, for by being there they keep away other and possibly harmful microbes.

On the other hand, some of these commensal organisms, such as *Staphylococcus pyogenes* which lives in the nose and on the skin, or *Streptococcus viridans* which lives in the mouth and throat, are potentially pathogenic. If the host's resistance becomes lowered they may produce disease. The balance between the pathogenicity of the microbe and the resistance of the host is a delicate one, and is easily upset. For example, in certain ill-defined 'run-down' conditions, *Staphylococcus pyogenes* living on the skin may start to invade the hair follicles, giving rise to a boil or carbuncle. One of the functions of the white blood cells is to prevent bacteria from invading the body. In the rare disease agranulocytosis, in which there are very few white blood cells, bacteria which normally live on the surface and are kept away from the internal tissues by these cells may start to invade, causing disease.

Another less dangerous type of staphylococcus, *Staphylococcus albus*, is also found in the nose and on the skin. An organism called *Neisseria catarrhalis* is commonly found in the throat and respiratory passages and is almost completely harmless. The bowel invariably contains large numbers of **Coliform bacilli** (*Escherichia coli*), which are harmless so long as they stay inside the bowel but can be extremely dangerous if they make their way elsewhere in the body, or if they are accidentally introduced, for example by an injection needle.

Carrier state

Sometimes, after recovery from an illness, people continue to be infected with the organism that caused it, and may transmit this organism to others, giving them the disease. Such 'carriers' are obviously a danger to the community. The best known example of this is that after an attack of typhoid fever, in which typhoid bacilli are present in the blood stream and the bowel, patients may continue to excrete the organisms in the urine and in the faeces. Obviously, if such people handle food or drink for others, there is a danger of infection. Outbreaks of typhoid can usually be traced to unsuspected carriers who have contaminated food.

There are many other examples of this 'carrier state'. Sometimes people who are immune may carry an organism without getting the disease; none the less, they are a danger to others. During poliomyelitis outbreaks there is always a large number of people living in the vicinity of a case of poliomyelitis who carry the virus in the bowel and excrete it in their faeces; their faeces may therefore carry poliomyelitis infection. When diphtheria was more common than it is today, children often carried the bacillus in their throats and infected others with it. Again, many people are unsuspected carriers of the hepatitis (jaundice) virus, which lives in the blood-stream. A syringe or needle can carry hepatitis virus from one person to another. This is one reason why it is important to use a sterilised syringe and needle whenever an injection is performed.

The effect of environmental factors

These may affect the incidence of infectious disease in a number of ways. Obviously, the more pathogenic bacteria there are in the environment, the more infectious disease there is likely to be. Some factors make for increased numbers of bacteria in the environment. For example, a high temperature may permit the breeding of flies which carry faecal microbes, or mosquitoes which carry malaria and yellow fever. Bad disposal of sewage and garbage will permit the multiplication of rats, which carry typhus and plague. Low temperatures discourage the multiplication of all microbes.

Paths of Infection

How do humans become infected with disease-producing microbes? The most important paths are the following:

1. *Infection through the Skin and Mucous Membranes*

The unbroken healthy skin is a good barrier against infection. This barrier is not merely a mechanical one, for the secretions of the skin have some bactericidal properties. These can be demonstrated by painting various kinds of bacteria on the skin and leaving them there. Bacteria which are not normally resident in the skin will mostly be killed within a few hours.

On the other hand, there is a normal resident flora of the skin which cannot be eliminated by washing with disinfectants. This consists largely of bacteria of low pathogenicity such as *Staphylococcus albus*, though pathogenic staphylococci are also often present.

Microbes, including the resident staphylococci, may penetrate the skin by way of the hair follicles or sweat glands, or through any abrasion or injury to the skin.

Pimples and septic spots in the skin are caused by the multiplication of staphylococci in hair follicles and in the dermis. **Boils**, caused by *Staphylococcus pyogenes*, nearly always start as infections in hair follicles. **Carbuncles** are boils which have joined together, producing a large mass of staphylococcal infection in the skin.

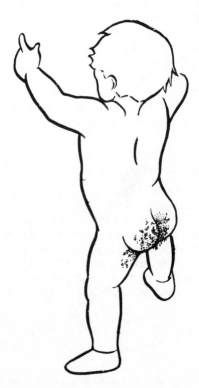

Fig. 15. The napkin area is particularly liable to infection

Almost any type of damage to the skin will lead to the multiplication of bacteria in it and hence to clinical infection. This damage may be through mechanical injury, or from some disease such as eczema or an allergic dermatitis. Burns, cuts, abrasions, and wounds of all kinds readily become infected. So do areas of roughness or chafing, or allergy. The larger the injury or abnormal area of skin, the more liable it is to infection. Excessive moisture from any source is a factor which may damage the skin and make it more liable to infection. This happens when perspiration accumulates in the body flexures, such as the skin underneath the breasts, between the toes, the perineum, and the axillae. Staphylococci, streptococci, and ringworm fungi are often the cause of infections in these sites. Soaked nappies, if neglected, often lead to serious infection of the skin of babies, which may become ulcerated and a source of great danger.

Moisture may also damage the skin of the hands, leading to clinical infection. This often happens at the sides of the fingernails, in those whose occupations cause them to immerse their hands regularly. Thus housewives, kitchen workers, fishmongers and bartenders are particularly liable to this type of skin disease. 'Chapped' hands are always likely to become infected.

People may infect their own skin from their noses, mouths, and throats, and also from the anus. Obviously, people may easily infect their own faces and mouths from their hands, hence the eyes, the nose, the respiratory tract and the gut may become infected.

Transmission of microbes from one person to another may occur by direct contact. In this way, usually through the hands, microbes from the skin, respiratory tract, eyes or gut of one person may reach the skin, respiratory tract, eyes, or gut of anyone with whom he is in contact. This

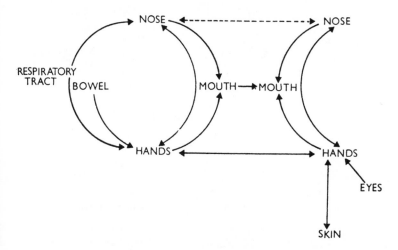

Fig. 16. Some possible sources of infection by direct contact

is the way in which many diseases may be spread, such as staphylococcal and streptococcal infections, rubella and measles.

Fungus infections of the skin are often picked up by contact from the environment, such as the infected floor of a changing room or swimming bath, or from infected clothing. These infections may be transmitted to other people by direct contact.

The **Mucous Membranes** are less resistant to infection than the skin, and nearly all have a numerous resident flora, Kissing may transmit any infection present in the mouth or respiratory tract. The venereal diseases, syphilis and gonorrhoea, are also transmitted by direct contact.

2. *Wound Infection*

The skin is the body's natural barrier against infection. When it is damaged, the underlying tissues are obviously liable to become infected from the environment. All wounds in which the continuity of the skin is broken may be infected from outside. Not only accidental wounds but surgical wounds may become infected.

Infection may occur (a) *At the time of the wound.* This may be from the microbes normally present on the wounded person's skin, or from his clothing. It may come from the instrument, missile or vehicle causing the injury, or from dust on the floor or in the air at the time.

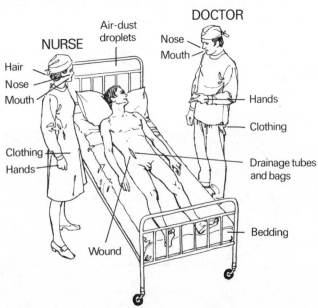

Fig. 17. Some possible sources of wound infection in a hospital

(b) *After the wound.* This may be from dust or air infecting the exposed tissues. In the case of surgical wounds, it may occur from instruments used for the dressing, from the dressings themselves, from the hands or respiratory tracts or skin of nurses or surgeons inspecting the wound. It may soak through damp dressings from the outside.

Not every microbe alighting on a wound causes infection. If the wound is bleeding freely, the mechanical action of the blood may wash the bacteria away. Anaerobic bacteria such as the gas gangrene and tetanus bacilli can only multiply in the absence of available oxygen; they are not likely to cause trouble in purely surface wounds. However, few traumatic injuries are confined to the surface.

Very many different types of bacteria can cause wound infection, and any exposed tissues may become infected. Moreover, the bloodstream may become infected giving rise to septicaemia.

Staphylococci, streptococci, *E. Coli, Pseudomonas aeruginosa* and *Proteus* are all common causes of wound infection. Anaerobic organisms also may be implanted deep into the tissues, together with dirt or fragments of clothing which will provide the chemical environment in which they can multiply.

3. *Infection from the Air*

This can occur either from infected droplets of respiratory secretion from a carrier, or from infected dust.

(a) *Droplet infection*

Droplets of secretion from the mouth, the throat, and the respiratory tract can carry microbes which may be inhaled by other people and so cause infection. All violent respiratory movements such as sneezing and coughing cause the expulsion of a shower of droplets from the mouth and nose. Shouting and talking also cause droplets to be ejected. These droplets may come from anywhere in the respiratory tract, from the nose and

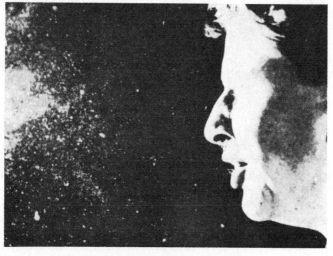

Fig. 18. Flash photograph of a cough

mouth to far down the bronchi. Everyone has experienced the odd droplet from a vehement talker.

Droplets vary in size. They consist of respiratory secretion and mucus, and contain bacteria from the part of the body from which they arise. As soon as the droplets enter the air, the fluid in them starts to evaporate. The smaller the droplets, the greater the rate at which evaporation will occur, as small particles have a relatively large surface area from which evaporation can take place. As the particles evaporate they get still lighter, and from the very smallest ones the fluid evaporates completely, leaving minute solid 'droplet nuclei' which are extremely light. These nuclei may be wafted long distances in air currents, carrying infection with them. Droplet infection may thus spread long distances, though this is rather unusual and the greatest danger is to those nearest to the infected person.

The larger droplets, on the other hand, fall to the ground almost immediately, only a few feet at most from the person expelling them.

Examples of diseases spread by droplet infection are numerous. Bacterial infections include pneumonia, tonsillitis, diphtheria, meningococcal infections and pulmonary tuberculosis. Virus infections include very common diseases such as colds, influenza, measles, rubella (german measles), and poliomyelitis.

It follows that patients with any of these infections which are spread by droplets are a danger to other people in their vicinity. Such patients should do all they can to limit the spread of infection from themselves, by covering their mouths and noses when they cough or sneeze, and by avoiding shouting or even loud talking.

Acute tonsillitis is caused by the *haemolytic streptococcus* which is almost always transmitted by droplet infection from the throat. This organism may also cause scarlet fever, otitis media, and broncho-pneumonia, any of which may result from droplet infection. Puerperal fever is also due to the haemolytic streptococcus and may result from infection of the birth passages from the nose or throat of the obstetrician or midwife.

Diphtheria was once a common danger from droplet infection. The bacillus was often 'carried' by healthy children and transmitted to others. Though the disease remains as serious as ever, its incidence has been enormously reduced by the widespread immunisation campaigns and carriers are now rare.

Colds are now known to be due to any one of a large number of different viruses which live in the mouth and nose, and infect other people by droplet infection. **Influenza** is also due to viruses, and is transmitted in the same way. Droplet infection is also probably the most important means of transmitting measles and rubella.

Pulmonary tuberculosis is usually transmitted by droplet infection. The tubercle bacillus is a waxy tough bacillus which can live for a long time in droplets. Cases of 'open' tuberculosis may cough the organism out in their sputum. All such 'open' cases are infectious, and no one should be allowed anywhere near them who has not been vaccinated against tuberculosis. On no account should unimmunised children be allowed in the same room as a case of suspected tuberculosis. Indeed, they should not live in the same premises if this can be avoided.

(b) *Dust infection*

Bacteria of various kinds can be carried in the air in dust. Staphylococci, *E. coli, Pseudomonas aeruginosa*, and the spores of tetanus and gas gangrene may all be carried about in dust, and may transmit disease when they land on the surface of human beings or are inhaled by them. This type of infection is important in hospitals, where there is usually a high concentration of many types of pathogenic bacteria. Air disturbance in hospitals may spread infection about.

Staphylococci from the skin may be shed into the air from clothing, and hence infect other people, making them into carriers or giving them disease. This is particularly dangerous in hospitals, where staphylococci are among the most important disease-producing microbes. This is because, more than most other pathogenic bacteria, they have the capacity to develop resistance to antibiotics. The majority of staphylococci found in hospitals are resistant to ordinary penicillin, though not, fortunately, to some of the newest types of penicillin. They are also often resistant to tetracycline and to other 'broad-spectrum' antibiotics, that is to say, antibiotics which are effective against a wide variety of different kinds of bacteria. Staphylococcal infections may therefore arise in patients who are being treated by these drugs.

Staphylococci are also possible causes of infection in operation wounds, either at the time of operation or later if the wounds are exposed for dressing or inspection in the wards.

Staphylococci and other bacteria may also enter the air in dust from bedding, ward curtains, cushions, and mattresses. During bedmaking rounds, the air of hospital wards is always found to contain more bacteria than at any other time. No dressings or aseptic procedures, such as venepunctures and lumbar punctures, should be done in wards until the dust from bedmaking has had time to settle.

Dry dirt from people's shoes and clothes may turn into dust and be drawn through the hospital by air currents. In this way, bacteria may travel through open doors, through the cracks around closed doors, up and down lift shafts, and into ventilation systems. This infection may reach into operating theatres, particularly if these are ventilated by extraction fans which draw in air from other parts of the hospital.

It has been shown that more patients get infected during operations if there is much bustle and coming and going in the operating theatre. In an experiment in one hospital, people were forbidden to enter or leave the operating theatre during operations. This measure alone reduced theatre infections to a fraction of what they were before.

Superficial lesions such as burns or operation wounds are especially liable to troublesome infections by air-borne bacteria. Patients with these lesions must be carefully protected. The lesions must not be exposed unnecessarily. Newborn infants in nurseries are also extremely susceptible.

Anything sterile which is exposed to the air in a hospital for any length of time, such as a bowl of sterile water, or a tray of dressings or instruments, is liable to be contaminated by air-borne infection.

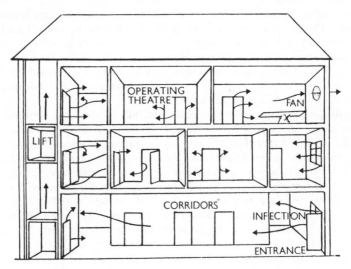

Fig. 19. Routes of infection within a hospital building

While vegetative bacteria, that is to say, those which do not form spores, can to some extent be controlled by the use of disinfectants in hospital, it is difficult to kill spores in this way. Only by rigidly avoiding the spread of dust can infection by the spores of gas-gangrene and tetanus be prevented. This means frequent washing of walls, floors, ceilings, and furniture, or dry-cleaning using vacuum cleaners. Spores from the air may not only fall upon the patient, giving rise to infection directly. They may fall upon opened drums or boxes of dressings, on instruments, into bowls of 'sterile' water, even into bowls of antiseptic solution which may be strong enough to kill 'ordinary' or 'vegetative' microbes but not spores.

Nearly all the infections spread by droplet nuclei mentioned in the last section may also be spread by dust. So may fungus spores, particularly those which cause infections of the respiratory tract. The dried droppings of birds and animals also become converted into dust and may be a source of infection.

Q fever, a rare form of pneumonia, is also spread by the air. This disease is caused by a rickettsia, a kind of large virus.

4. *Infection from Food and Drink*
Any microbes which are passed in the stools are liable, when hygienic conditions are poor, to contaminate food or water, and so transmit

infection. Many types of infection are spread in this way. These include the salmonella infections, which are typhoid and paratyphoid and infective food-poisoning. Typhoid and paratyphoid are sometimes called the 'enteric' diseases. Dysentery, cholera and many virus infections such as polio and hepatitis are also spread in this way (see Chapters 5 and 6).

The contamination is usually indirect. The microbes reach the food or drink either via the hands of infected people, or by the soiling of the hands with infected faecal materials, or by being carried by flies or other animals.

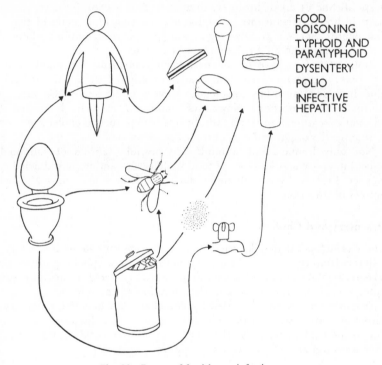

FOOD
POISONING
TYPHOID AND
PARATYPHOID
DYSENTERY
POLIO
INFECTIVE
HEPATITIS

Fig. 20. Routes of food-borne infection

In **salmonella infections**, the bacilli are excreted in the patient's faeces, which are highly infective and dangerous. After recovery, patients may continue to excrete bacteria in their faeces for long periods. This is most likely to happen in a patient with a chronically infected gall-bladder, particularly if this contains gallstones.

In the **'enteric'** fevers, typhoid and paratyphoid, the organisms may also be found in the patient's blood-stream, and they may be excreted in the urine. This may continue after the patient has recovered from the disease, and a urinary carrier can contaminate water supplies. This happened in a serious typhoid outbreak in Croydon in 1936, when a urinary carrier of typhoid bacilli infected a reservoir, causing over 300 cases of typhoid and many deaths.

Many people in the past have recovered from typhoid but have continued to 'carry' the bacilli, and such people, if they are engaged in the preparation of food, may transmit the infection. 'Typhoid Mary' was such a case. She was a typhoid carrier who worked as a cook in New York under various false names, moving from post to post in households and institutions. During this time she infected thousands of people, and caused many deaths from typhoid. She refused to give up her work, but years after she was first recognised as a carrier she was caught and detained in hospital. She escaped, however, and worked as a cook for several more years in hotels, restaurants and sanatoria, causing more cases of typhoid and deaths. She was finally caught and placed in detention, where she remained until she died twenty-three years later.

Similar carriers have in the past been responsible for many serious outbreaks of typhoid. They should never be allowed to prepare or handle food intended for other people, and every effort should be made to eliminate the infection. Nowadays, most carriers can be cured by antibiotic treatment, or if this fails, by operations, such as cholecystectomy, to remove the organ which is chronically infected.

Not only humans but animals are possible sources of salmonella infection, as are certain types of food such as eggs and imported dried egg powder. Processed vegetable foods, such as dried coconut, have also been sources of infection.

Dysentery and Cholera

The dysentery bacilli, like the salmonellas, are spread in the stools of sufferers from the disease. As with typhoid and paratyphoid, patients who have recovered from the illness may continue to excrete the bacilli for some time. Faecal contamination and flies may spread the infection.

Dysentery may also be caused by amoebae, and amoebic dysentery is common in tropical countries. **Cholera**, a very acute disease of the bowel due to the cholera bacillus, also occurs in most tropical countries which have an unreliable or unsafe water supply.

Food Poisoning from Bacterial Toxins

Some bacteria form a toxin when they multiply in food. If the food is then consumed without being heated sufficiently to destroy the toxin, the consumers may develop food poisoning. **Staphylococci** are the commonest cause of this, and staphylococcal enterotoxin may develop in any food that has been carelessly handled by people with staphylococcal lesions of the hands. *Clostridium welchii*, the gas-gangrene bacillus, is another microbe which produces a toxin and may give rise to food poisoning in this way.

Infection of Foods of Animal Origin

Foods of animal origin may carry pathogenic bacteria from the animals. Thus, **milk** from tuberculous cows was formerly an important source of infection, resulting in tuberculosis of the lymph-nodes, bowel, bones and joints, and tuberculous meningitis. These diseases have now been eliminated from some countries by excluding tuberculous cattle from dairy herds. In this country and in several others, all milk is now obtained from 'T.T.' (tuberculin tested) herds which are known to be free from tuberculosis.

Brucellosis (undulant fever) is an infection transmitted in the milk and milk products of cattle which still occurs in country districts. **Streptococcal** infection from streptococcal mastitis of cows may also be transmitted in this way. Both these diseases may be prevented by pasteurising the milk.

Eggs and **dried egg powder** as possible sources of salmonella infection have already been mentioned.

Alimentary Virus Infections

Some virus infections are also spread by contamination from the faeces. The most important is **poliomyelitis**. The polio virus lives in the gut, and may be spread by contamination from the faeces, directly from humans or indirectly by flies. It may also be spread by droplet infection from the mouth. During poliomyelitis outbreaks, many healthy people carry the virus and may spread it to others.

Infective hepatitis (virus jaundice) is another virus disease which may be transmitted in this way.

5. *Infection from the Soil*

The soil contains bacteria dropped in the faeces of cattle. The richer the soil in manure, the more infective it is. Almost any rich garden or farm soil contains many of these bacteria.

The most dangerous of these microbes are the bacilli of gas-gangrene (*Clostridium welchii*) and of tetanus (*Clostridium tetani*). These bacteria form resistant spores which can survive adverse conditions, including extremes of temperature. They are **anaerobic**, that is to say, the spores germinate and the bacteria multiply only in the absence of oxygen.

These organisms may produce disease when they infect deep wounds with a poor blood supply. In such wounds they can multiply, causing disease which may be fatal if not promptly treated. Garden injuries, even if apparently trivial, have been known to lead to tetanus—for example, pricks with rose thorns. Another dangerous kind of injury is that sustained by the gardener who digs a fork through his boot and into his foot.

Road accidents, war injuries, and indeed almost any kind of wound may lead to gas gangrene or tetanus.

The bacilli of gas-gangrene and tetanus are found often in the bowel of human beings. Intestinal obstruction, which may lead to the escape of these microbes from the bowel into the peritoneal cavity, may also give rise to Clostridial peritonitis.

Anthrax is a cattle disease caused by a spore-bearing bacillus which may also be found in the soil in the neighbourhood of infected cattle. This is dealt with more fully in the next section.

6. *Infection from Animals*

Domestic animals, pets, cattle and insects may all carry pathogenic microbes. Perhaps the commonest types of disease spread by cattle are fungus diseases of the skin and scalp such as 'Ringworm'. The spores of these fungi may spread directly from person to person, by direct or indirect contact. As has already been mentioned, infected cattle may spread disease microbes in their **milk**. Tuberculosis, brucellosis, and streptococcal infection may all be spread in this way.

All domestic animals, and pets such as tortoises and birds, may spread salmonella infection from their faeces, giving rise to food poisoning or enteric fever.

Anthrax is a disease of cattle due to a spore-bearing bacillus. The bacillus is aerobic; that is, it can multiply only in the presence of oxygen. The spores may be transmitted to human beings from the hides, hairs or fur of cattle, causing serious infection which begins in the skin but soon spreads to the bloodstream. The spores may also be present in the dust of wool processing works, and may be inhaled by the workers giving rise to a dangerous form of pneumonia known as 'wool-sorters' disease'. As might be expected, this disease used to be common in Yorkshire.

Human anthrax is often a mortal disease, though fortunately it can usually be controlled by antibiotics. In order to reduce the risk of anthrax infection, all imported hides and furs are required by law to be sterilised before they are released to factories or shops for processing or sale.

Rats are responsible for many types of serious infection throughout the world, such as plague. This disease is carried to man by rat fleas. It is endemic in some of the great overcrowded cities of the East. The Great Plague of 1665 in London was the last serious outbreak in Great Britain.

Endemic typhus is another disease spread to humans from rats by rat-fleas. Like plague, it occurs in big overcrowded cities which are infested by rats. It is a different disease from **Epidemic typhus**, which is spread by lice from one human being to another. Both types of typhus are due to rickettsias (see page 82).

Rats may also spread **Weil's disease**, or infectious jaundice. This is due to a spirochaete called *Leptospira icterohaemorrhagica*, which is excreted in the urine of the rat. Weil's disease is found in people who are in close contact with rats. It used to be common among fishworkers in Dundee and other towns in Scotland where fish was processed in rat-infested open sheds by the water front. It is also found among sewage workers, and in people who live in damp rat-infested basements. Occasionally, people get infected by falling into canals. Dogs may transmit a variety of Weil's disease, but this is vary rare.

Even more rare, but exceedingly dangerous, is **rabies**. This may be spread not only by infected dogs but by other carnivorous animals, such as wolves, and numerous cases in the United States have been shown to be due to bats. It is an acute disease of the nervous system, and is spread by the bites of the infected animals, in whose saliva the virus is present.

Rabies became extinct in Britain because of the rigid quarantine regulations imposed on the import of dogs and other animals from abroad. At the time of writing, there is some fear that it may be re-introduced owing to a breach of these regulations.

Dogs also transmit **toxocariasis**, due to a roundworm, *Toxocara canis*, which they excrete in their faeces. Human beings may become infected from dog faeces, and blindness is one of the possible results. Such infection is thought to be common owing to the widespread fouling of streets and public places by dog faeces.

Another disease spread by dogs, which may also take many forms including blindness, is **Toxoplasmosis**. This is due to a protozoon, *Toxoplasma gondii*, and is not to be confused with toxocariasis in spite of the similar name. Again the extent of human infection is not known for certain, nor is it known exactly how infection is acquired from dogs and possibly other animals.

Nearly all domestic animals are subject to salmonella infection, which causes a mild generalised disease in human beings. Dogs, cats, monkeys and tortoises have all been shown to transmit this type of disease. Often the animals themselves contract the disease from dirty pet shops, and bring it from there into the home.

Birds may transmit psittacosis, or parrot-fever, a form of pneumonia due to a variety of small bacterium called a chlamydia. Not only parrots but budgerigars and other birds have been responsible for this. Budgerigars have also, in rare cases, been shown to transmit polio.

Arthropods (insects and the like) transmit many types of pathogenic microbe. **Flies**, which feed indiscriminately on human food and on sewage, transmit all types of faecal infection. They can spread typhoid, paratyphoid, dysentery, food-poisoning, trachoma, polio and hepatitis. Plague is carried from rat to rat by fleas, and human beings may contract it by being bitten by infected fleas. **Murine** or **Asiatic typhus** is carried in the same way. **Epidemic** or **classical typhus** is spread from man to man by the bites of infected lice. Various other kinds of typhus found in different parts of the world also have an arthropod intermediate host which carries the disease to man. Thus, in North America, there is a tick-borne disease called 'Rocky Mountain Spotted Fever'. Another type of typhus found in the Pacific region of Asia, is transmitted by mites. **Yellow fever**, an acute hepatitis found in Central Africa and Central and South America, is a virus disease spread by the bite of a mosquito. Vaccination against this infection is essential for anyone planning to stay in the infected zone. A large number of different viruses cause **encephalitis** (brain inflammation) in different parts of the world; they too are spread by mosquitoes.

The commonest arthropod-borne disease in the world is **malaria**. The malarial parasite is a protozoon, spread by the bites of mosquitoes.

CHAPTER 4

THE CONSEQUENCES OF INFECTION

What happens when a human being becomes infected with a pathogenic microbe depends on a large number of factors, which may be considered as either:

(a) **Host Factors** — The **Soil** on which infection is sown.

1. *The effect of environment*

Environmental factors play a large part in determining the resistance of the individual human being to infection. In general, resistance is directly related to the standards of living. Where these are lowest, infectious disease is most common. This is particularly true of such epidemic diseases as cholera and plague, which are never entirely absent from the poor and overcrowded cities of the Far East. It is also true of tuberculosis, in which there is a very marked association with standards of living. Tuberculosis is essentially a disease of overcrowded or undernourished communities. The problem of infectious disease is greatest in communities with inadequate sanitation and health services. Such communities are very much at the mercy of their environment which is largely uncontrolled. Bad water supplies, rats, flies and mosquitoes are the chief causes of infectious illness; these are aggravated by poor housing and nutrition, and by ignorance of the elementary principles of hygiene.

In certain infections, of which poliomyelitis is the most notable, living standards affect the incidence in a complicated way. A rise in standards not only lowers the total incidence but also raises the age at which people are likely to contract the disease. Thus, in poor countries, poliomyelitis is a disease mostly of children — 'infantile paralysis'. In richer countries, relatively more adults and less children get the disease. This is because the disease is largely spread by faecal contamination and sewage. In poor countries, children are more likely to become infected owing to bad hygienic conditions, and hence to develop the disease, or to become immune to it from contact. In richer countries they are likely to be protected in early years, but they fail to develop immunity, owing to lack of contact with the virus.

2. *The site of infection*

The microbes may hit upon a part of the host in which they are incapable of causing disease. Thus influenza viruses are only dangerous if they enter the respiratory tract. On the skin, or in the bowel, they are harmless. The spores of Clostridia can cause disease only if they are in a deep wound. They too are harmless on the skin or in the bowel, in which they are, in fact, often found.

However, many microbes are invasive, that is, they have properties

32

which enable them to travel in the body of the host and multiply in various tissues. Virulent staphylococci, streptococci and *E. coli* can all cause disease in a variety of situations in the human body. Tubercle bacilli, in susceptible subjects, can multiply in various sites — in the lungs, in the gut, on the skin and so on. The spirochaete of syphilis can do likewise as can anthrax bacilli and other virulent bacteria. The viruses of smallpox and measles enter the body through the mucous membrane of the respiratory tract. They multiply in that site and travel to various other sites before they reach the skin, where the greatest multiplication takes place.

The response of the host to infection depends on his or her state of **immunity**. This itself depends on a complex series of factors, and is dealt with in detail in Chapter 10. Some of these factors are specific, that is, they relate to resistance to particular microbes. Others are non-specific, that is, they relate to resistance to microbes as a whole.

In the early stages of microbial disease the commonest form of response by the body is that known as **inflammation**. The form which this takes differs in different parts of the body. However, it is worth considering the implantation of *Staphylococcus pyogenes* into the skin as typical of the inflammatory process in general.

Staphylococci usually gain entry into the body through the base of a hair follicle. This is situated in the dermis, or corium, beneath the protective epidermis. The microbes start to multiply in the corium and as they do so they produce various toxins. The most important of these are **leucocidin**, which damages the white cells and may kill them, **necrotizing toxin**, which kills various cells, **haemolysin**, which destroys red blood cells, **coagulase**, which clots fibrinogen, and **fibrinolysin** which has the opposite effect, and dissolves clots.

These toxins act in various ways to help the proliferating microbes to establish themselves, though the precise mechanism is not known so far as all of them are concerned. Thus, coagulase, by clotting plasma, protects the microbes from the action of leucocytes. Fibrinolysin, by breaking down clots, helps the organisms to spread along blood vessels. Leucocidin damages the leucocytes and impairs their phagocytic powers. The formation of a wall of fibrin around the proliferating microbes is the most characteristic feature of clinical staphylococcal infections such as boils and carbuncles, which tend to be localised. At the same time, the host's defences go into action to try to localise and combat the infection. Polymorph leucocytes migrate to the site of invasion via the blood stream.

The entry of many more leucocytes than usual into the blood stream is the reason why, in the early stages of an infection, there is a higher white cell count than normal. This **leucocytosis** is a feature of all such infections, and its detection by means of a white cell count is, in fact, an indication that a 'pyogenic' infection is taking place. This is why the doctor often asks for a white cell count to be done in a patient in whom infection is suspected. As virus infections usually do not produce a leucocytosis, this test may serve to differentiate bacterial from virus infections.

Inflammation is one of the most obvious signs of disease, and its main features were recognised in ancient times as **heat, swelling, redness,** and **pain**. These are always present at the site of an inflammatory lesion, and may readily be seen even in a trivial inflammation in the skin.

The heat and redness are due to the increased blood supply to the affected part. The swelling is due partly to this, and partly to the exudate of body fluid in the actual lesion. Pain is a result of the swelling, for distension of any part of the body, particularly against pressure, is one of the most important causes of pain.

Pus. The function of the polymorph leucocyte is to ingest and destroy microbes. This process is called **phagocytosis**. The leucocidin produced by the microbes damages the leucocytes. So the infection at this stage takes the form of a battle between the polymorphs and the bacteria. 'Pus' consists of a collection of live and dead leucocytes and bacteria in such an infective process, which is often known as a 'pyogenic' (pus-forming) infection. Put in another way, 'pyogenic' infections are those in which the polymorph leucocytes of the blood are stimulated.

If the host is well immunised against this particular type of infection, he readily produces antibody to the microbe (see Chapter 10). The antibody sticks to the outside of the microbe and attracts the polymorph chemically to it, so that the microbe is more readily ingested. This is known as the 'opsonic' effect — the antibody or 'opsonin' makes the microbe more palatable to the leucocyte. The Greek word 'opson' means a seasoning or sauce. In his play *The Doctor's Dilemma*, Bernard Shaw described the process through the mouth of his character Sir Colenso Ridgeon:

'The phagocytes won't eat the microbes unless the microbes are nicely buttered for them. The patient manufactures the butter for himself.'

A vigorous response on the part of the body defences to invasion by pyogenic organisms usually results in their localisation and death, and in rapid recovery from infection. This response depends on a number of factors. One of these is the ability of the bone marrow to produce large numbers of polymorph leucocytes when required. In leukopenia or agranulocytosis, which may be caused by certain poisons and drugs, the ability to produce leucocytes is impaired and the patient is unable to respond to bacterial invasion by a brisk leucocytosis. Such patients may therefore become seriously ill on account of an infection which would be trivial in a normal person.

The modern treatment of certain diseases by immunosuppressive drugs artificially reduces the patients' resistance to infection. These patients also are at special risk of infection.

Another factor is the ability of the tissues to respond, by increased vascularity and so on, to the need for increased circulation of blood to the infected part. Yet another is the need for rapid production of antibody. Both of these essential parts of the inflammatory response are to some extent controlled by the secretion of the adrenal cortex. Excessive secretion damps down the response, as does the administration of cortical hormones such as cortisone and prednisolone. Patients under treatment with these drugs are less well able than the normal person to produce an inflammatory response when needed.

(b) **Parasite Factors**

Some bacteria are not pathogenic at all, others are highly pathogenic. The differences in pathogenicity are due to a number of factors which are closely related. To some extent, however, they can be sorted out, and the following are the most important:

1. **Infectivity**. The capacity of the organism to spread from one host to another.

2. **Toxigenicity**. The capacity to produce toxins which damage the tissues of the host. Examples are diphtheria toxin and the various toxins of the staphylococcus mentioned earlier in this chapter.

3. **Invasiveness**. The capacity to invade the tissues of the host, and to multiply and spread within them.

The word **virulence** is also sometimes used to mean the combination of toxigenicity and invasiveness.

The above terms are all rather vague, and there is no common agreement about the precise meaning of any of them. None the less they are useful concepts if they are used broadly, in a commonsense way. For example, a bacterium may have a high infectivity but a low virulence. In this case, it would give rise to a high carrier rate, but little illness. If infectivity were low but virulence high, the organism would produce **sporadic** cases of disease (see page 36).

An example of a factor affecting infectivity is the way in which some types of cell attract certain viruses. Thus, the influenza viruses attach themselves to the cells of the mucous membrane of the respiratory tract; having done this, they can easily gain entry into these cells and cause disease.

The production of toxins is perhaps the most obvious factor making for pathogenicity. However, toxin-producing bacteria, such as the diphtheria and tetanus bacilli, differ widely in the amounts of toxin they produce under specified conditions. Another important point is that the pathogenicity of a particular type of bacterium varies from time to time. The factors which cause these variations have been much studied, and a good deal is known about them. For example, virulent strains of most types of bacteria can be made non-virulent by growing them under artificial conditions in the laboratory. When this happens, the microbes lose certain characteristics which account for their virulence. Thus, when they are infecting an animal, pneumococci have slimy capsules surrounding them. They lose their capsules when they are cultured in the laboratory. Similarly, many toxin-producing organisms gradually lose the capacity to produce toxin when they are cultured in artificial media.

On the other hand, inoculation into animals or infection of human cases usually make an organism more virulent than it was before. This change may also be accompanied by a morphological change. Thus, in the tissues, the pneumococcus regains its capsule which is associated with virulence.

Such changes as these can be regarded as responses to different environments. On a culture plate in the laboratory, life is easy for the microbe. There is plenty of food and there are no enemies, and it can multiply without having to contend with such adverse factors as leucocytes and antibodies. It does not need such a complicated chemical structure, such a complex armament of toxins and so on, as it does when it is trying to establish itself in the tissues of a living host. So its chemical structure is simplified accordingly under artificial conditions. When it enters an animal host, on the other hand, the microbe has to fight for survival against the cells and body fluids of the host which do their best to kill it. In these circumstances the microbe needs to produce toxins and other agents of chemical warfare if it is to have any chance of surviving.

One important consequence of this increase in virulence after passage through animals or human beings is that the intensity of an infection may increase during the course of an epidemic as the microbe passes from one human or animal to another. This also accounts for the relatively high virulence of microbes in the hospital environment, where there is a continuously changing population of susceptible people in whom the microbes can maintain their virulence.

Epidemiology: Sporadic, Endemic and Epidemic Disease

Infections are said to be **sporadic** when occasional cases occur in a community, without any spread. These infections are usually those of low infectivity, which need rather special conditions to establish themselves. Thus tetanus is nearly always a sporadic infection.

Diseases may also become sporadic when populations acquire a high degree of immunity. Thus diphtheria, which used to be endemic in this country, is now sporadic as most people are immunised against diphtheria early in life.

An infection is **endemic** when it is constantly present in the community, increasing and diminishing in intensity at various times but never dying out completely. Most infections which regularly occur in this country are endemic, such as staphylococcal and streptococcal infections, and virus diseases like measles, chickenpox, and mumps. In overcrowded cities with large and uncontrolled rat populations, murine typhus and plague, in which human beings are infected from the rats, are often endemic. The infections are never completely eliminated from the rats and are always liable to spread to humans.

The actual incidence of an endemic disease at any particular time depends on a balance between several complicated factors. The relative numbers of immune and susceptible people is one of these; another is the relative virulence and invasiveness of the organism, which also varies continually.

An **epidemic** is the word used to describe an outbreak of disease in which a large number of people become infected within a short time, and infection continues to spread throughout the community.

Epidemics may occur in communities who have never met that particular type of infection before. Such groups of people are usually very susceptible, and disease may spread through them like wildfire and be extremely virulent. Missionaries and traders from populous countries may bring epidemics to isolated areas. Thus a community in Greenland suffered a devastating outbreak of measles some years ago; the fatality rate was very high because the population had never been in contact with measles before and had no resistance to it.

An unfamiliar infection such as typhoid may also become epidemic when a single carrier is allowed to spread organisms to an unprotected community owing to some breakdown in hygiene. This occurs from time to time in European countries which are normally free from typhoid.

Infections which are usually endemic may become epidemic in particular circumstances. Thus an epidemic of staphylococcal infection may occur in a surgical ward of a hospital if the aseptic technique of the operating theatre or of the ward staff is inadequate. A single carrier of staphylococci may spread the infection to a number of surgical patients, from whom it may spread to other members of the staff and hence to other patients. Such an epidemic may spread through many wards and cause much trouble.

Epidemics may start up very quickly. Influenza outbreaks spread rapidly in towns and at their height may involve the majority of the population. Cholera is another example. If the water supply of a town becomes infected with the cholera bacillus, the number of cases may rise very sharply indeed in a few days.

An epidemic usually goes through a definite cycle in which the numbers of cases of the disease increases up to a peak and then begins to fall of its own accord. This is because the number of susceptible people is limited. After they have all become infected there are none left to continue spreading the infection. It is possible today to stop many infections by serological means or by antibiotics. Thus in a poliomyelitis outbreak in a city in the north of England, the mass immunisation of the population stopped the epidemic in its tracks. Some bacterial epidemics can also be stopped by the administration of antibiotics in small doses to the whole population, thus breaking the chain of infection between carrier and susceptible person.

CHAPTER 5

THE MAIN TYPES OF INFECTIVE ILLNESS— *BACTERIAL INFECTIONS*

Staphylococcal Infections

Staphylococci are gram-positive cocci which form clusters which look, under the microscope, rather like bunches of grapes (see Fig. 14).

The most pathogenic types of staphylococci are called *Staphylococcus pyogenes* or *Staphylococcus aureus.*

The course of events in a typical staphylococcal infection was outlined in the last chapter. The special feature is the formation of a fibrin wall or 'core' in the lesion.

Staphylococci are often found in the noses of healthy people, whence they spread to the skin and all over the body. These organisms are, moreover, peculiar in that they are more liable than any other types of microbe to develop resistance to antibiotics.

The toxins produced by staphylococci in the tissues are listed on page 33. The commonest type of staphylococcal disease is skin infection. This takes the form of pimples, septic spots, impetigo, boils, and carbuncles. Unhealthy, macerated, or broken skin is also liable to become infected by staphylococci; these organisms are the commonest causes of minor sepsis in grazes, cuts and burns. Staphylococci not only cause superficial infections, however; they may enter the blood stream and cause disease in many parts of the body, such as osteomyelitis, perinephric abscess and subphrenic abscess. Staphylococcal pneumonia is a common and dreaded consequence of infection in post-operative patients. It may lead to empyema. Otitis media and meningitis may also be caused by staphylococci; indeed, suppuration may occur in any organ.

Staphylococcus albus is a type of staphylococcus which is usually harmless and which is often found on the skin and in the nose of normal people.

Laboratory Diagnosis

Superficial or discharging lesion:
Examination of swab or pus (collected in sterile container)—

1. Microscopy of stained smears.
2. Culture and sensitivity tests.

Swabs should not be left lying about for hours before they reach the laboratory as they are liable to dry up. They should never be incubated or placed in a refrigerator. On the other hand, staphylococci may remain alive for many hours on a swab at room temperature. If some delay is inevitable before the swab can be handled, because of the hour at which it is taken or the distance from the laboratory, it may still be possible to grow staphylococci from it. As with all pathology specimens, the swab must be correctly labelled at the time it is taken with the patient's full name, the ward, the date, and the type of specimen. Endless trouble results from the incomplete labelling of swabs.

Some laboratories issue special 'transport media' in which the swab can be placed and left safely for hours before examination. This is particularly useful in places where the laboratory is some distance from the hospital; it is also helpful for general practitioners.

In some cases in which there is no discharging lesion, the following tests may aid the diagnosis:

Blood culture. This is a valuable test in suspected septicaemia, in which the organisms multiply in the blood stream. A blood sample is taken by venepuncture under aseptic conditions to prevent contamination of the specimen. The blood is immediately expelled from the syringe into bottles of culture medium. About 10ml of blood should be taken. Blood cultures are rarely positive unless the patient has a raised temperature at the time. It is worth waiting for a rise in temperature before the specimen is taken.

Blood count, particularly a white cell (leucocyte) count. A leucocytosis suggests an active pyogenic infection (see page 33).

Phage-typing. When *Staphylococcus pyogenes* has been isolated, the strain of the organism may be determined by the **phage** (or **bacteriophage**) **typing** technique. There are many types of staphylococcal phages, which are viruses which destroy or **lyse** staphylococci. Staphylococci can be classified into strains according to the types of phage which lyse them. In this test, the culture of staphylococci isolated from the patient is treated on a petri dish with suspensions of different phages. Next day the plate is examined, to see which types of phage have lysed the staphylococci. This gives the strain of the staphylococcus; for example, if the lysing phages are types 80 and 81, the staphylococcus is strain 80/81, and so on.

Some phage types are more pathogenic or more invasive than others. In an outbreak of staphylococcal infection, ascertaining the phage types of all the staphylococci isolated may enable the source of the outbreak to be traced.

Antibiotic Treatment

In hospitals today, the majority of staphylococci are resistant to ordinary types of penicillin. Many strains are also resistant to tetracycline and to other antibiotics. Staphylococcal infection is therefore often relatively difficult to treat. It can be a serious menace in hospitals, and indeed, it is one of the most important types of infection to be found within hospitals, since most other types can easily be controlled by antibiotics.

The reason why most types of penicillin-resistant staphylococci are able to resist this antibiotic is that they produce an enzyme, **penicillinase**, which destroys penicillin.

Some modern varieties of penicillin, such as Methicillin (Celbenin) and Flucloxacillin are not destroyed by penicillinase and are therefore active against staphylococci resistant to ordinary types of penicillin.

The choice of antibiotic should always be guided by the result of sensitivity tests. These are performed by placing various antibiotics on a culture plate on which the organisms are growing to see which antibiotics inhibit their growth. The antibiotics may be applied to the culture plate in the form of filter papers impregnated with solution, or of tablets containing the drug. Alternatively, holes may be cut in the plate and filled with solutions of the antibiotic, which then diffuses into the agar.

Prevention

1. **The control of carriers**. Nasal carriers and skin carriers should be detected by swabs. If *Staphylococcus pyogenes* grow from the swabs they should be phage-typed to determine their strain. Nasal carriers should then be carefully treated with a suitable nasal cream or spray.

Hand carriers can be controlled by the use of antiseptic soaps such as hexachlorophene soaps, or 'phisohex'.

2. **The protection of vulnerable patients**. Nurses, students, doctors and domestics with superficial staphylococcal infections should never be allowed into surgical wards, operating theatres, maternity units or infants' nurseries.

All surgical wounds should be kept covered by sterile dressings. If the dressings have to be taken down for any reason, this should only be done under full aseptic precautions.

Newborn infants are also especially liable to pick up staphylococcal infections. Sterile gowns should be put on and hands should always be washed when babies are to be lifted. Fresh clean medicaments and ointments should be used for babies. The less the babies are handled, the better.

Women in labour should be treated as if they were surgical cases undergoing operations.

Streptococcal Infections

Next to staphylococci, streptococci are probably the commonest cause of pyogenic infections. They, too, are gram-positive cocci. Under the microscope they are seen to form chains (see Fig. 14).

The most pathogenic type of streptococcus is called *Streptococcus pyogenes* or the haemolytic streptococcus.

In infections due to this organism, there is little localisation on the whole, in contrast to staphyloccocal infections. The infection tends to spread throughout the body.

Haemolytic streptococci produce many toxins, of which the most important are **Haemolysins**. These destroy red blood cells, and are responsible for the clearing effect of the organism seen on blood agar plates. Other toxins are as follows:

Streptokinase, which digests fibrin and thus helps the organisms to spread throughout the body. **Hyaluronidase** increases the permeability of the tissues and has a similar effect in spreading infections.

Erythrogenic toxin causes the red rash on the skin in **scarlet fever**, which is a type of streptococcal sore throat accompanied by a rash.

Acute tonsillitis is the commonest disease caused by streptococci. Steptococci may also cause puerperal fever, otitis media, cellulitis, meningitis, and acute inflammation in any other part of the body. In septic abortions, the infecting organism is often a haemolytic streptococcus.

Streptococci may also have serious delayed effects, due to **allergy** on the part of the host. Streptococcal allergy is due to an abnormally high antibody production. The most important of these effects is the development of **acute rheumatic fever** some weeks after the streptococcal illness. This is a dangerous disease in children and young people. It is chiefly dangerous because it may lead, after many years, to crippling heart disease. Mitral stenosis, in which the mitral valve becomes thickened and partly closed, is one of the end results. Older people may get a more chronic type of rheumatism affecting one or two joints, or rheumatoid arthritis. Another late result of haemolytic streptococcal infection is acute nephritis or Bright's disease. This too may progress to chronic disease of the kidney.

A type of streptococcus which is often harmless is *Streptococcus viridans*. This is usually found in the mouth and throat of normal people. It may, however, produce a serious infection of the heart valves of people with congenital abnormalities or old rheumatic infection of the valves, giving rise to 'subacute bacterial endocarditis'.

Streptococcus faecalis is a common and normal inhabitant of the bowel. It is non-haemolytic and does not alter the blood on culture plates.

Strep. faecalis is a frequent cause of urinary infections. It may also cause abscesses, particularly in the perineal region, pneumonia, and suppurative infection anywhere in the body. It is an occasional cause of subacute bacterial endocarditis.

Laboratory Diagnosis

Examination of swab or pus.
1. Microscopy of stained smears.
2. Culture and sensitivity tests.

Pathogenic streptococci are subdivided into a number of groups called 'Lancefield' groups. When a streptococcus is cultured from a specimen therefore, the group to which it belongs may be found by a further laboratory test. The most dangerous haemolytic streptococci belong to Lancefield Group A. These are the organisms most often associated with rheumatic fever and nephritis. Groups C and G are also occasionally found in acute streptococcal infections. *Streptococcus faecalis* belongs to Lancefield Group D.

Blood culture in suspected septicaemia, and in suspected subacute bacterial endocarditis. In suspected rheumatic cases, an examination of serum for antistreptolysins (streptococcal antibodies) may be useful.

Antibiotic Treatment

Penicillin is the first choice. All haemolytic streptococci are sensitive to it, and *Strep. viridans* is usually sensitive. However, *Strep. faecalis* is occasionally resistant.

Sulphonamides and tetracyclines are also effective.

Prevention

Suspected carriers should have throat and nasal swabs taken. If positive, they should be treated with pencillin.

It is a common practice for the staffs of maternity wards to have regular throat swabs to detect streptococcal carriers and hence to minimise the danger of puerperal sepsis.

Recurrences of rheumatic fever often follow haemolytic streptococcal infections. These may be prevented, in rheumatic patients, by small daily doses of pencillin or sulphonamides. Children who have repeated tonsillitis may have to have their tonsils removed.

Pneumococcal Infections

Pneumococci are sometimes regarded as a variety of streptococci. They often cause lobar pneumonia in adults or bronchopneumonia in children, and they may also give rise to a severe type of meningitis. If left untreated, pneumococcal infections give rise to a characteristically thick greenish pus.

Laboratory diagnosis

Examination of swab, pus, or sputum.
  1. Microscopy of stained smears — the organisms are gram-positive, lance-shaped, and are found in pairs ('lanceolate diplococci').
  2. Culture.

Antibiotic Treatment

Penicillin is the first choice. Sulphonamides and tetracyclines are also useful.

Prevention

The disease is of low infectivity and preventive measures are of little value.

Neisseria Infections

Neisserias are a group of organisms which include two important pathogens, the gonococcus, which causes gonorrhoea, and the meningococcus which causes acute meningitis. They are gram-negative cocci, kidney-shaped, and usually found in pairs, hence they are sometimes called diplococci.

Gonorrhoea

Gonorrhoea is a venereal disease. Infection is spread by direct contact from the urethra of the man to the cervix of the woman, or vice versa. This disease is an acute inflammation, with a purulent discharge in which the gonococci may be found. They appear as pairs of kidney-shaped gram-negative organisms inside the pus cells.

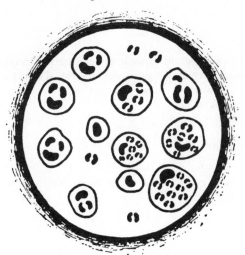

Fig. 21. Smear of gonococcal pus, showing diplococci. The large blobs inside the cells are the cell nuclei; the small ones are the diplococci

In the early, acute stage the treatment of gonorrhoea is fairly simple both in men and women. Most cases respond to antibiotics. However, it is essential for success that treatment be started early. In *women*, the infection may spread rapidly to the fallopian tubes, giving rise to inflammation (salpingitis). This is perhaps the commonest cause of sterility in women. In *men*, untreated or inadequately treated gonorrhoea may lead to chronic infection of the urethra, which after many years may become fibrous, and develop a stricture. The patient finds it difficult to pass urine, and may eventually be quite unable to do so without catheterisation.

Infection with the gonococcus always results in disease; it is impossible to develop immunity to this organism. An individual exposed to infection may have frequent attacks.

Laboratory diagnosis

(a) Examination of fresh discharge, taken:

In men, from the urethra, after cleansing the meatus.

In women, from the cervix or urethra. A vaginal speculum should be used to locate the cervix and urethra. Vaginal swabs are of little value as the organism is readily killed by the acid content of the vaginal wall.

1. Microscopy of stained smears shows the characteristic gram-negative intracellular diplococci.

2. Culture of the organisms, which are not easy ones to grow, and sensitivity tests. In both sexes, the organisms may occasionally be isolated from the rectum or throat. Swabs should be cultured *at once*. If this is not possible, they should be broken into a suitable transport medium, and kept at room temperature until they can be cultured. Organisms should survive for up to 24 hours.

(b) **Blood tests**

In all cases, especially those with disseminated infection or of long standing, the serum may show a positive Gonococcal Complement Fixation Test (G.C.F.T.). However, false positives also occur, owing to cross-reaction with meningococci.

Antibiotic treatment

Penicillin is the first choice. A single dose of 1-2 mega units of procaine penicillin cures most cases in the acute stage. Tetracycline and erythromycin are also effective.

Prevention

The only sure prevention is avoidance of sexual intercourse with infected people.

Meningococcal Infections

There are many causes of acute meningitis, which is always a dangerous disease. The *meningococcus* is one of the most important of these. Meningococcal meningitis is an epidemic disease, and the organism is spread by droplet infection. Outbreaks occur in overcrowded communities such as barracks. During an outbreak many carriers are found who harbour the organism in their nose or throat, and may transmit it to others. Some of these may develop catarrhal symptoms; in others, the organism travels from the nose to the central nervous system and causes meningitis. Occasionally meningococci may give rise to septicaemia which may be extremely acute and is often fatal.

Laboratory Diagnosis

In all suspected cases of meningitis, **lumbar puncture** is performed as diagnosis is impossible without an examination of the spinal fluid.

1. Microscopy of stained smears. The meningococcus looks like the gonococcus and appears as a gram-negative intracellular diplococcus.

2. Culture and sensitivity tests.

Antibiotic treatment

Most cases respond readily to penicillin and sulphonamides, but some meningococci are resistant to sulphonamides.

Prevention

The prevention of overcrowding, especially of sleeping quarters, diminishes the risk of infection.

Other Neisserias

Various organisms, of which *Neisseria catarrhalis* is the most common, are found in the mouth, nose and respiratory tract of most normal people, in whom they do not cause disease. Under the microscope they look like gonococci and meningococci.

Haemophilus Infections

Haemophilus influenzae

This is a slender gram-negative bacillus. It is often found in the respiratory tract, where it may cause sinusitis, chronic bronchitis, or bronchopneumonia. It is also one of the most important causes of meningitis in childhood. At one time it was thought to be the cause of influenza, but this is now known to be a virus.

Laboratory diagnosis

In respiratory infections: examination of pus or sputum.
In meningitis: examination of spinal fluid obtained by lumbar puncture.

1. Microscopy of stained smears.
2. Culture and sensitivity tests.

Antibiotic treatment

First choice: Ampicillin.
Second choice: Tetracyclines.

Klebsiella Infections

Klebsiella pneumoniae (Friedlander's bacillus)

This is a gram-negative bacillus which may cause secondary infection of the respiratory tract, giving rise to sinusitis, chronic bronchitis, or bronchopneumonia. It may also cause urinary infections, especially in catheterised hospital patients.

Coliform Infections

The colon bacillus, *Escherichia coli*, is a gram-negative, flagellated and motile rod. It is usually a harmless inhabitant of the bowel. Occasionally it gets into other organs such as the urinary tract, where it may cause acute pyogenic infection. *E. coli* is much the commonest cause of urinary infections — cystitis, pyelitis, or pyelonephritis. It may also cause pneumonia and suppuration anywhere in the body. Some varieties, or strains, of *E. coli* may also cause gastro-enteritis, particularly in residential communities such as hospitals and nurseries. These are called 'entero-pathogenic' or 'atypical' strains.

Laboratory Diagnosis of urinary infections

A fresh clean **mid-stream specimen of urine** should be obtained. Passing a catheter is dangerous as it may itself cause a urinary infection. The urine should be cultured and the centrifuged deposit examined unstained under the microscope. The presence of pus cells and organisms indicates infection. In doubtful cases, the organisms or cells may be counted, using special methods. A number of kits for culturing the urine are now available commercially.

Antibiotic treatment

Co-trimoxazole, kanamycin, ampicillin, sulphonamides, tetracyclines, furadantin or other antibiotics.

E. coli is not sensitive to penicillin.

Salmonella Infections

A large group of bacteria called the Salmonellas resemble *E. coli* in that they are gram-negative flagellated bacilli. However, they are all pathogenic and cause disease of the small bowel. The most important are the typhoid and paratyphoid bacilli which cause typhoid and paratyphoid (enteric) fever. Other types of salmonella, of which there are several hundreds, cause acute bacterial food poisoning. The methods of spread of these infections is dealt with in Chapter 3.

Typhoid and Paratyphoid

Typhoid and paratyphoid are acute and serious diseases which start 7-10 days after swallowing the microbes. The main feature is infection of the small bowel, producing diarrhoea which may become chronic. This may lead to perforation of the bowel, a dangerous complication. In addition, other parts of the body may become affected when the organisms invade the bloodstream, which occurs early in the disease.

After recovery from infection the patient may continue to excrete the bacilli in the stools and become a chronic 'carrier'. This is most likely to happen in people with gallstones, in which the organism may lurk for years. Patients with renal stones may likewise become urinary carriers, and continue to excrete the organism in the urine.

Laboratory Diagnosis

In early stages: Blood culture.
In all stages: Culture of the faeces and urine.
After 10 days of illness: examination of the serum for antibodies (Widal reaction).

Antibiotic treatment

First choice: Chloramphenicol.
Second choice: Amoxycillin or ampicillin.
Carriers: Faecal carriers should be treated with amoxycillin or ampicillin; if this is unsuccessful, cholecystectomy may be necessary.

Prevention

(a) General hygienic measures as for food-borne infections (see Chapter 8).
(b) Immunisation with vaccines. Three doses at intervals of about four weeks, by subcutaneous or intradermal injection.

Food Poisoning (see also Chapter 3)

(a) Salmonella food poisoning

In addition to the typhoid and paratyphoid bacilli there are hundreds of other species of salmonella. They are responsible for **acute bacterial food-poisoning**, an illness in which diarrhoea and vomiting start 12-24 hours after eating or drinking the infected food. Attacks usually clear up after a few days without special treatment.

The commonest cause of salmonella food-poisoning in this country is *Salmonella typhi-murium*, the mouse-typhoid bacillus. Another important cause is *Salmonella enteritidis*. Typhoid and paratyphoid bacilli do not usually cause this type of disease.

Laboratory diagnosis

Culture of organisms from stools and vomit, sometimes also from blood. If the suspicion falls on any particular item of food, this should be cultured if possible.

Detection of antibodies in blood 10 days or more after the onset.

Antibiotic treatment (usually not necessary)

Ampicillin or chloramphenicol.

Prevention

As for food-borne infections in general (see Chapter 8).

(b) **Toxic food-poisoning**

Some bacteria, if they are allowed to multiply in food, produce a toxin in the food. If this is subsequently eaten, an acute food poisoning may follow within a few hours, usually less than 12 hours. *Staphylococcus pyogenes* is the commonest cause of this type of poisoning.

A moderate room temperature is sufficiently high for these organisms to multiply and produce dangerous quantities of enterotoxin. The toxin is relatively resistant to heat, and is not destroyed by temperatures which will kill the organisms themselves. Cooking will not necessarily make the food safe once toxin has been formed in it. Food suspected of being infected should therefore be thrown away.

It is most important, therefore, that food should not be allowed to be contaminated by staphylococci or clostridia, and that it should not be allowed to stand about for long periods at room temperature but should be kept covered and in a refrigerator (see also Chapter 8).

Staphylococcal poisoning is one of the commonest varieties of food poisoning. Most attacks, however, are not reported to a doctor, and it is often impossible to trace the exact cause, as it is no easy matter to detect staphylococcal toxin in food even if any of the food is available for examination, which is not often the case.

This type of poisoning is due to swallowing an already formed toxin, not to swallowing bacteria. The mechanism is therefore quite different from that in salmonella food poisoning, which is due to the actual multiplication of microbes in the small bowel. **Antibiotic treatment** is useless.

Clostridium welchii may produce a similar disease, apparently by multiplying in the bowel and producing toxin there. Food infected with *Clostridium welchii* spores is therefore dangerous.

Dysentery

This is an illness in which the patient suffers repeated attacks of diarrhoea, often with the passage of blood and mucus in the stools. At the start of the disease there is also often a general illness with a rise in temperature. There are two main varieties of dysentery, **bacillary** and **amoebic**. Bacillary dysentery is caused by the Shigellas, a group of gram-negative bacilli which resemble the salmonellas except that they have no flagella and are not motile. There are many types of dysentery bacilli which are common in all countries where food hygiene is bad. The commonest ones are the Sonne and Flexner dysentery bacilli. The commonest cause of amoebic dysentery is *Entamoeba histolytica.*

Laboratory Diagnosis

Bacillary dysentery: Microscopy and culture of the stools.

Amoebic dysentery: Microscopy for amoebae. A fresh specimen is best and it has to be warm for the motile amoebae to be detected. In older specimens the characteristic cysts may be recognised.

Treatment for Bacillary Dysentery

First choice: Sulphonamides. Either soluble sulphonamides such as sulphadiazine, or insoluble ones like succinysulphathiazole, may be used. The latter have to be given in very large doses.

Second choice: Ampicillin or Tetracyclines.

Treatment for Amoebic Dysentery

Metronidazole; emetine compounds.

Prevention

As for food-borne infections in general (see Chapter 8).

There is no effective form of immunisation against dysentery.

Cholera

The cause of cholera is a curved bacillus with a single flagellum at the end, called *Vibrio cholerae.* It is gram-negative and motile, and can easily be cultured on ordinary media.

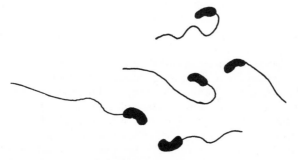

Fig. 22. Cholera vibrios

Cholera is perhaps the most acute and serious of the food-borne bacterial infections. It occurs in overcrowded cities with a poor water supply. Outbreaks are liable to occur in any part of the world. A feature of these is that large numbers of people contract the disease almost simultaneously, which places a great strain on the medical and public health services. Moslem pilgrim ships have occasionally suffered outbreaks and any mass pilgrimage in the East is a possible focus.

The disease has an incubation period of three to five days, after which the diarrhoea and vomiting begin. The mucous membrane of the small intestine becomes intensely inflamed. Large patches of it flake off and are passed out in the motions. Dehydration is the greatest danger, and the usual cause of death. If this can be controlled by parenteral therapy, the patient will probably survive.

Laboratory Diagnosis

Demonstration of vibrios in stained smears from stools.
    Culture of vibrios from stools.

Treatment

Treatment of dehydration. Antibiotics such as tetracycline and furazolidine may also be of value.

Prevention

Control of food and water supplies.
    Immunisation: One or two doses of cholera vaccine for primary immunisation. A single dose for subsequent visits to cholera areas. Immunity lasts for only 3-6 months after the injections.

Proteus and Pseudomonas Infections

Proteus mirabilis (formerly called B. proteus) is a gram-negative bacillus, normally found in the faeces, which often causes wound infection and infection of the urinary tract. It has two features which make it extremely troublesome. First of all, it is very motile. It multiplies rapidly on a culture plate spreading quickly or 'swarming' across the plate as it does so. The second troublesome feature is its resistance to many of the usual antibiotics.

Another similar organism is called *Pseudomonas aeruginosa*. This bacterium also grows in a 'swarming' fashion. It produces a green-blue pigment known as 'pyocyanin' which may colour the pus it infects. Like Proteus, *Ps. aeruginosa* is often a difficult infection to treat by ordinary methods. Both of these organisms may spread rapidly from one case to another in hospitals. They may contaminate instruments such as catheters, and pseudomonas has been found in the dust of hospital wards. It may even be found in 'antiseptic' solutions.

Laboratory Diagnosis

Culture of organisms from fresh stools.

Antibiotic treatment

Local: Neomycin and polymyxins.
Systemic:
  Ps. aeruginosa: Polymyxins, such as thiosporin or colistin, gentamicin
          or carbenicillin.
  Proteus: A suitable antibiotic should be determined by sensitivity tests.
          Carbenicillin, kanamycin, co-trimoxazole and streptomycin
          are often effective.

Brucellosis—Undulant Fever

Brucella abortus and *Brucella melitensis* are relatively small gram-negative
bacilli which occasionally cause a variety of septicaemia called 'Undulant
fever'. They are found in cattle and goats, and human beings are infected
from the milk of these animals. The disease mostly occurs in country
districts where milk and cream are not pasteurised. It is also common in
Mediterranean countries. 'Malta fever' is a variety of Brucellosis.

Human infection by brucella is often difficult to diagnose. Many people
have only a trivial illness which is regarded as an attack of influenza. The
clinical features of a typical attack are persistent fever with few physical
signs, and do not suggest any particular type of illness in the early stages.
The fever fluctuates, with alternate periods of rise and fall of temperature
over several days, hence the term 'undulant fever'.

Laboratory Diagnosis

1. Blood culture. The organism may take several weeks to grow.
2. Detection of antibodies in the serum, after two weeks or more of
illness.
3. Skin test for allergy to 'Brucellin', an extract of brucella organisms,
may be useful in cattle. In man, it is unreliable, as a positive result may be
due to past infection.

Antibiotic treatment

Tetracyclines are the most effective drugs, preferably with sulfadiazine or
streptomycin.

Prevention

Pasteurisation of milk and cream.

Diphtheria

Diphtheria is due to a gram-positive bacillus of slender and often irregular or granular shape called *Corynebacterium diphtheriae*. This organism reaches its usual site, the back of the throat, by droplet infection.

Here it multiplies in the susceptible subject, producing its toxin which damages the cells of the mucous membrane, giving rise to a fibrinous exudate. This clots and forms a membrane on which the organisms continue to multiply. They produce more toxin which gets into the blood stream and circulates throughout the body causing damage especially to the heart, kidneys, adrenals and peripheral nerves. The tissues of the neck become acutely inflamed and swollen, producing the characteristic 'bull-neck' of diphtheria. Occasionally infection may occur in the nose instead of the throat; this is 'nasal diphtheria'.

The diphtheria bacillus is dangerous because of the toxin it produces, and the disease is due to the action of the toxin. If the toxin is neutralised by antitoxin, no illness occurs. If the infected subject is immunised so that he is able to form his own antitoxin he will not become ill when he is infected (see Chapter 10).

Laboratory Diagnosis

Culture of organisms from a throat or nasal swab. This may take up to 48 hours, and special selective media have to be used.

As some strains of the diphtheria bacillus are not pathogenic, pathogenicity is always confirmed by tests for the production of toxin. This is necessary also because there are many organisms, called 'diphtheroids', which resemble the diphtheria bacillus but are harmless, and are often found in the throat and on the skin.

Treatment

Antitoxin with penicillin.

Diphtheria is a killing disease and it is important that the treatment of a suspected case should not be delayed. It should be started as soon as there are good grounds for suspecting diphtheria, without waiting for the laboratory report. The dose of antitoxin ranges from about 2000 units in a mild case in a small child to 50 000 units or more in a severe case in an adult.

Contacts of cases who have not been actively immunised should be protected by injections of 500-1000 units of antitoxin after a susceptibility test (see below).

Prevention

Diphtheria is a good example of an illness which can be prevented by 'active immunisation'. The value of immunisation is clearly shown by statistics of the incidence of diphtheria and the number of deaths due to this disease, before and after the immunisation campaign had started in Great Britain.

Until widespread immunisation started in 1940, approximately 40 000-50 000 people developed diphtheria every year, of whom about 2000 died. Most of these were young children. The incidence rate and the number of deaths fell very rapidly until in the last few years diphtheria has been a rare disease in Britain.

There can be no doubt that every child born in this country should be actively immunised against diphtheria at an early age. Immunisation against whooping cough and tetanus can also be given in the same series of injections, using a combined preparation (see Chapter 10). It is possible to combine poliomyelitis immunisation in the same dose, but separate oral administration is probably a more effective way of immunising against poliomyelitis.

Antitoxin is prepared from the serum of immunised horses. This is liable to give rise to allergic reactions in a proportion of human subjects, and these reactions may be quite serious. A test dose to detect susceptibility should always be given before antitoxin is administered (see Chapter 10).

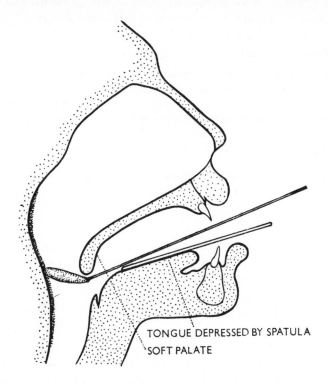

TONGUE DEPRESSED BY SPATULA
SOFT PALATE

Fig. 23. Taking a post-nasal swab

On the other hand, toxoid which is used to give active immunisation is almost harmless. This is another very good reason for giving active immunisation early in life, followed by a booster dose at about five years of age.

Pertussis (Whooping Cough)

The **whooping cough bacillus** (*Bordetella pertussis*) is the cause of one of the most serious infections of early infancy. It is gram-negative. The organism is inhaled and settles on the mucous lining cells of the trachea and bronchi, where it multiplies. After an incubation period of 7-10 days the disease begins with a 'catarrhal' stage, resembling a heavy chest cold. Then after a few days the characteristic paroxysms of coughing may occur repeatedly and are extremely exhausting to the patient, who is usually a small child.

The chief danger of pertussis is that it may be complicated by broncho-pneumonia or lobar pneumonia, and it is as a result of these diseases that death may occur.

While in the typical case it may be easy to diagnose whooping cough on clinical grounds, in some cases the whoop is only occasional and may be thought to be due to some other type of respiratory disease.

Laboratory Diagnosis

Culture of organisms from a throat swab, per-nasal swab or post-nasal swab. A per-nasal swab is taken by pushing a swab gently through the nostril to the nasopharynx. A post-nasal swab is a bent swab which is put into the mouth and swabs the pharynx behind the soft palate (see Fig. 23).

Antibiotic treatment

This is of doubtful value in mild cases. Ampicillin or chloramphenicol in serious cases.

Prevention

Vaccination in infancy. Some children have developed encephalitis after vaccination, but most experts agree that the risk is small and less than that of contracting pertussis if the child is not vaccinated.

Tuberculosis

The **tubercle bacillus** (*Mycobacterium tuberculosis*) is a slender, slight, irregular, rod-like organism with a waxy coat which is water-repellent. This makes it difficult to stain. Hot concentrated stain has to be used, and once the organism is stained the stain cannot be dissolved out by acid or alcohol. The bacillus is, therefore, said to be 'acid and alcohol fast'. In medical conversations, the expression 'A.F.B.' (acid fast bacillus) is often used instead of 'Tubercle bacillus', particularly when there is any danger of a conversation being overheard by the patient or his relatives. Another euphemism is 'Koch's bacillus', so called because the organism was discovered by Robert Koch.

There are two main varieties of tubercle bacillus. The **human** bacillus causes disease in humans only, and is mostly spread by droplet infection. The **bovine** organism causes disease in cattle as well as human beings. It may also be spread to humans in the milk of infected cattle.

Tuberculosis occurs all over the world. It is commonest where living standards are lowest, that is in the great cities of the East and the industrial areas of Western cities. Some varieties of tuberculosis, such as pulmonary tuberculosis, are very infectious, and overcrowding favours infection. Outbreaks may, therefore, occur in closed communities such as the crews of ships and inmates of mental hospitals, and prisons. The disease also occurs and spreads in lodging houses and in slum dwellings.

It is, however, important to realise that tuberculosis can be almost completely prevented by methods which are widely used. These are the immunisation of susceptible people and the isolation of known cases of active disease. So far as bovine tuberculosis is concerned, the elimination of infected cattle from dairy herds, so that their milk can no longer spread infection to humans, is the best method. If this is impracticable however, as it is in many poor and developing countries, the milk should be pasteurised. In this process the milk is heated to a temperature, usually between 60° and 75° C, at which the tubercle bacilli are killed. Pasteurisation has greatly helped to reduce the incidence of tuberculosis in many countries.

Improvements in the general standard of living, especially in nutrition and housing and the avoidance of overcrowding, are also important factors in reducing the incidence of tuberculosis.

It is quite easy to find out which members of the population are susceptible and which are immune. Susceptible people can be immunised by means of BCG (see page 58). Infectious cases of tuberculosis can be isolated, and kept under surveillance after they have recovered.

Infected cattle can be detected by tuberculin testing. In this country, as in many others, only milk from tuberculin tested ('TT') herds is allowed to be used for human consumption.

As a result of these measures tuberculosis is well on the way to extinction in this country, and has been much reduced in all parts of the world. The bovine disease has almost completely disappeared from Great Britain and several other countries.

After infection with the tubercle bacillus, the disease is slow to develop. It may affect any part of the body, and destroys the healthy tissues. The lungs are most commonly attacked; this is **pulmonary tuberculosis**. In this form of the disease the lung tissue is gradually destroyed and breaks down, so that cavities form within the lung. From these the patient may cough up large numbers of tubercle bacilli into his sputum, which may then spread to others by droplet infection. This is the most important way of spreading the disease. Such a patient with 'open' pulmonary tuberculosis is a serious danger to all susceptible people who should be kept well away from him. The patient should be isolated in a single room if possible; he should certainly not be nursed in a general ward. He must be educated to understand the danger of his sputum droplets flying about. He must be taught to cover his mouth with his hand when he coughs; after coughing he should wash his hands in disinfectant solution which is kept covered. Disposable sputum pots should be used, which are carefully disinfected before being thrown away.

A similar discipline must be used in the dressing of tuberculous wounds, such as those of sufferers from bone or joint tuberculosis, or tuberculosis of the lymph nodes. This type of disease is now rare in Britain and several other countries because the main cause, the bovine tubercle bacillus, has been removed by eliminating tuberculin-positive cattle from dairy herds.

Laboratory Diagnosis

Demonstration of the tubercle bacillus from suspected material:

1. Microscopy of smears stained by special methods such as the 'ZN' (Ziehl-Neelsen) and auramine methods.

2. Culture and sensitivity tests.

3. Guinea-pig inoculation.

As the organism is not always seen in smears, culture or guinea-pig inoculation should be performed in every case. Guinea-pigs are extremely susceptible to tuberculosis and will always develop the disease if infected material is injected into them. Cultural methods, however, are almost as reliable and are much less expensive.

Sensitivity tests of the organism against anti-tuberculous drugs should also be performed to guide the treatment.

Smears may be examined within a few hours, or, preferably, minutes, of taking the specimen. Cultural and inoculation tests, however, may take several weeks to show a result as the organism grows very slowly.

Allergy and Immunity (see also Chapter 10)

Once they are infected with tubercle bacilli people develop **allergy**; their tissues become sensitive to the tubercle bacillus. The result is that if they become infected with tubercle bacilli for a second time their tissues react with local inflammation and necrosis. This reaction occurs not only after infection with living tubercle bacilli but after contact with killed organisms or with extracts such as tuberculin.

Allergy is accompanied by *immunity*. An allergic person, that is, one who has already been infected at some time in the past, is immune to further infection. All who have recovered from tuberculosis, or who have had a subclinical infection — one so mild that they have not been ill at all — are immune, and can, therefore, be permitted to be in contact with cases of open tuberculosis with relative safety. If we find that a person is allergic, this also means that he is immune. By doing tests for allergy on a group of people, or a whole population, therefore, it is possible to differentiate them into the immune and the non-immune. Like most types of immunity this is not absolute; it is possible for an allergic person to develop tuberculosis, but this is uncommon.

The tests for allergy consist of introducing into the skin an extract of tubercle bacilli such as tuberculin or 'PPD' (Purified Protein Derivative of tuberculin). This may be done by the intradermal injection of measured quantities — the **Mantoux** test; or by 'firing' with a 'gun' of sprung needles — the **Multiple puncture** or **Heaf** test.

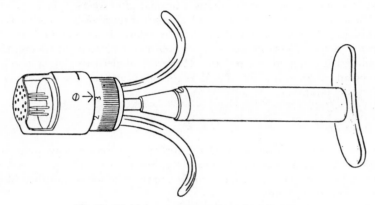

Fig. 24. Multiple puncture gun for tuberculin tests

The Mantoux test is the most exact, and permits the injection of known amounts of varying concentrations of tuberculin. It is usual to start with an injection of 0.1ml of 1/10 000 dilution (1 tuberculin unit). If the result is negative, one proceeds with 0.1ml of 1/1000 dilution (10 units). If this too is negative, 0.1ml of 1/100 dilution (100 units) is given. However, this test requires a separate syringe and needle for each patient and takes time; a group of patients cannot be tested quickly by a doctor working single-handed. The multiple puncture test is quicker and less expensive; it is probably the most convenient on the whole, especially when many people have to be tested at a single session.

All tuberculin tests should be read in 48 or 72 hours. If the result is positive, an area of erythema (reddening) and induration (thickening) occurs at the site of the application or injection of the tuberculin.

Treatment

Tuberculosis is a slow disease to develop, and it is also slow to cure. The modern treatment consists essentially of rest, and the use of anti-tuberculous drugs. There are numerous drugs active against the tubercle bacillus, of which the most used are streptomycin, para-amino-salicylic acid (PAS), isoniazid, and rifampicin. These are used in combinations of two or more drugs because if only one, or even two, drugs are used, the organism may acquire resistance to them. Tubercle bacilli may easily become resistant to streptomycin if it is used alone; in fact, they may even become streptomycin-dependent, that is, they may be unable to live without streptomycin.

Streptomycin is a rather dangerous drug; medication for long periods may lead to permanent deafness or damage to the vestibular nerve. The onset of this can be very insidious. The main symptom besides deafness is inability to balance properly; this may not become apparent in a bed-ridden patient until he starts walking about and even then it may be missed for some time as some unsteadiness is normal after weeks in bed.

The most difficult type of tuberculosis to treat successfully is tuberculous meningitis. A combination of all three standard drugs may be given by various routes. It may be necessary to continue treatment of tuberculous meningitis for four to six months. However, modern treatment is often successful whereas before the days of streptomycin the disease was invariably fatal.

Prevention

(a) General measures to avoid the spread of infection: environmental hygiene, the avoidance of overcrowding, the isolation of open cases of tuberculosis, the pasteurisation of milk, and the elimination of tuberculous cattle from dairy herds.

(b) The protection of the individual:
    1. Adequate nutrition, especially vitamin D.
    2. Immunisation.

Immunisation

Susceptible people can be vaccinated against tuberculosis by the injection of **BCG**. This procedure has an interesting history. Robert Koch discovered the tubercle bacillus in 1882, and soon afterwards made the first tuberculins, or extracts of tubercle bacilli. He considered that tuberculin might be used to immunise against tuberculosis, but this was shown to be wrong. However, many attempts were made to produce effective immunising agents against the disease. Killed vaccines were useless, and vaccines of live organisms were too dangerous. Then in 1906, two French bacteriologists named Calmette and Guérin started to prepare a vaccine. Their idea was to produce an attenuated vaccine, that is to say, one that was 'weakened' so that it would no longer produce disease, but could give rise to immunity against the fully virulent organism. This they rightly thought they could achieve by growing the organism on a very artificial medium. After many years, they succeeded in making the organism non-virulent, and it is now used for immunisation throughout the world (see also Chapter 10). BCG stands for 'Bacille Calmette-Guérin'.

Since the war BCG had been used on a wide scale, and it is now used in this country also as a means of immunising young people. It is given by intradermal injection. All who are likely to be in contact with cases of tuberculosis should be immunised, for example, medical students, nurses, and other hospital workers. Immunisation is now offered to all school-children at the age of 13, in Great Britain, and most take advantage of the offer.

When injecting BCG one gives the person a harmless 'primary' injection with tubercle bacilli. This confers allergy and immunity just as would an injection of the virulent organism, but without the dangerous effects of the latter.

In the years following BCG vaccination, the vaccinated person may well make his first natural encounter with the tubercle bacillus after contact with a case of active disease. If this happens, the immunity already received is strongly reinforced, and will probably last for the person's lifetime.

If possible, a tuberculin test should be previously performed on the person whom it is proposed to immunise. If the result is positive, BCG should not be given. To do so would not only be unnecessary, since allergy and immunity are present already, but dangerous as a troublesome reaction would probably follow.

BCG is given into the skin, usually on the side of the arm. A few days after the injection a small nodule appears at the site. This becomes vesicular, and the blister remains for some weeks, then gradually disappears. The whole cycle usually takes 6-12 weeks.

Leprosy

The leprosy bacillus, *Mycobacterium leprae*, is an acid fast bacillus related to the tubercle bacillus.

Leprosy is an age-old disease which has occurred in most countries of the world. Today its greatest incidence is in Central and other parts of Africa, Southern Asia, Southern Europe, and Central and South America. The mode of infection is not known but the disease has a low infectivity. It is possibly spread from the nasal secretions, as these often contain large numbers of organisms in typical cases. The incubation period varies a good deal but is always long and may be several years.

The disease is slow to develop and progresses over a period of years. There are two clinical types. In the **lepromatous** type masses of granulation tissue appear and there is much destruction of normal tissue. In the **tuberculoid** type the nerves are affected and sensation is lost. This is followed by muscular atrophy, and trophic lesions of the skin.

Laboratory Diagnosis

Microscopy of stained smears from the lesions, to demonstrate the characteristic slender, acid-fast bacilli occurring in clusters.

The organisms cannot be cultured in the laboratory.

Antibiotic treatment

Sulphone drugs, such as dapsone.

Anthrax

The **anthrax bacillus** (*Bacillus anthracis*) is a relatively large, gram-positive bacillus. It is aerobic and has the ability to form spores under adverse conditions (see Chapter 2). In culture, and in the tissues, it often produces long chains, which look under the microscope rather like bamboo sticks.

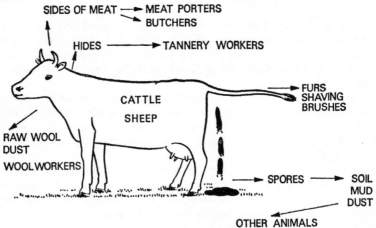

SIDES OF MEAT ⟶ MEAT PORTERS
BUTCHERS

HIDES ⟶ TANNERY WORKERS

CATTLE
SHEEP

FURS
SHAVING
BRUSHES

RAW WOOL
DUST
WOOL WORKERS

SPORES ⟶ SOIL
MUD
DUST

OTHER ANIMALS

Fig. 25. The Spread of Anthrax

The organism is found in cattle, and spores occur in the hides of animals. Human beings usually get infected from animal hides or from products of hides such as furs, shaving brushes, and the like. The disease anthrax has a marked occupational incidence; agricultural workers and meat porters are most often affected owing to their constant contact with sources of infection.

Anthrax may occur in any country but is rare in Great Britain. The usual form of the disease begins at the site of implantation of the organism as an acute infection of the skin which becomes inflamed, swollen and necrotic. This is called a malignant pustule, but it does not contain pus. The organisms may easily be demonstrated in the lesions at this stage. From the skin lesion the organisms enter the blood-stream, producing a septicaemia. This is often fatal in the absence of antibiotic treatment.

Laboratory Diagnosis

(a) Examination of swabs or pus or fluid from the lesions.
  1. Microscopy of stained smears.
  2. Culture and sensitivity tests.
(b) Blood culture.

Antibiotic treatment

Penicillin.

Prevention

Sterilisation of imported hides, furs, shaving brushes, etc. This is enforced by law.

Immunisation of farm animals.

Deep burial of infected animals; this prevents germination of spores.

Plague

The plague bacillus, *Yersinia pestis*, is a gram-negative, non-motile bacillus, which is found in the bloodstream and in the lymph nodes of sufferers from plague. It is the cause of an ancient scourge, the **bubonic plague** of which there have been large outbreaks periodically throughout human history. The Black Death of the fourteenth century was plague, and killed about 25 million people, or about one quarter of the population of Europe. Outbreaks have occurred in various places from time to time; the last big outbreak in England was the Great Plague of London in 1665.

Plague is a disease of rats which is carried to humans by fleas. It is, therefore, essentially a disease of overcrowded communities with large, uncontrolled rat populations. Like many other mass epidemic diseases it occurs most often in the great overcrowded cities of the East, in India, and the countries of South-east Asia. However, it is by no means confined to them, and outbreaks occur occasionally in Africa, America, and Europe.

The disease usually starts a few days after the bite of an infected flea. The organism spreads from the bite to the local lymph nodes which enlarge, becoming inflamed and then dusky—the 'buboes'. At the same time the patient becomes febrile and prostrated. The organisms enter the bloodstream and spread throughout the body; death occurs in about fifty per cent of cases unless effective antibiotic treatment is started.

There is also a pneumonic type of plague due to droplet infection from other cases. This is a rapid, severe, and often fatal disease.

Laboratory Diagnosis

Examination of material obtained by aspiration of lymph nodes or from sputum.

1. Microscopy of stained smears.
2. Culture and sensitivity tests.

Antibiotic treatment

Streptomycin and sulphadiazine.

Prevention

Control of rats and fleas.

Immunisation

By living or killed vaccines.

Clostridial Infections

Gas gangrene and **tetanus** are two diseases which are spread by spores (see Chapter 2).

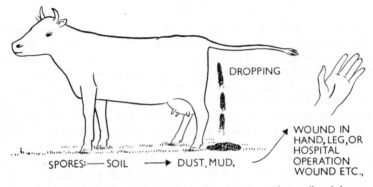

DROPPING

WOUND IN HAND, LEG, OR HOSPITAL OPERATION WOUND ETC.,

SPORES:—— SOIL ——→ DUST, MUD,

Fig. 26. The spread of gas gangrene and tetanus spores from soil and dust

The organisms which cause them are gram-positive bacilli which live in the bowel of man and animals, and reach the soil in the droppings of animals. Spores of tetanus and gas gangrene can easily be found in soil; they are also present in many kinds of dirt and they are carried about in dust. They can only germinate into the bacilli in anaerobic conditions, that is where there is little or no free oxygen or air.

Any penetrating wounds are liable to be infected with the spores of the gas gangrene and tetanus bacilli, particularly those in which much dirt, soil, clothing and so on is introduced. Compound fractures, in which dead fragments of bone may be left in the wound, are also dangerous. The wound does not have to be a large one to be dangerous, and quite trivial injuries have given rise to tetanus (see Chapter 3). Animal bites are also liable to lead to tetanus if they are not properly treated. The two diseases, gas gangrene and tetanus, are quite different clinically.

Gas Gangrene

Gas gangrene is usually due to *Clostridium welchii*; there are several other related organisms which may also cause the disease, of which the commonest are *Clostridium septicum* and *Clostridium oedematiens*. The spores of one or more of these organisms germinate in a deep or dirty wound, forming relatively large gram-positive bacilli. These produce exotoxins which damage the host cells, and may kill them. The bacteria migrate along the path of the dying cells and enter the bloodstream, producing a septicaemia. If untreated, the organisms may attack the muscle cells produing gas in the cells, hence the term 'gas gangrene'.

Clostridium welchii is a normal inhabitant of the gut. In cases of acute intestinal obstruction it may pass from the gut into the peritoneal cavity giving rise to a clostridial peritonitis. This is a very serious and often fatal condition. Infection of the perineal soft tissues may also occur after operations for rectal resection, or after colostomy operations. One of the toxins produced by *Clostridium welchii* is an enterotoxin, or small intestine poison. If food contaminated with *Cl. welchii* spores is eaten, the organisms may multiply in the bowel, producing enough toxin to give rise to food poisoning, a similar disease to staphylococcal food poisoning (see page 48).

Laboratory Diagnosis

Examination of swabs from wound:
1. Microscopy of stained smears.
2. Culture (clostridia are anaerobic).

If the wound is large several swabs should be taken from various parts of it.

Treatment

Surgical, combined with penicillin or tetracycline, and anti-gas gangrene antitoxin. Barrier nursing of cases is not necessary as *Clostridium welchii* is a normal inhabitant of the gut.

Prevention

Prophylactic penicillin and tetracycline, with antitoxin as soon as possible after the wound.

Tetanus

Clostridium tetani, the tetanus bacillus, does not spread through the tissues or invade the blood stream as does *Clostridium welchii*. The spores remain at the site of implantation where they germinate and multiply only if anaerobic conditions prevail, that is, in wounds with little blood supply or much dirt, debris, or dying tissue.

The bacilli secrete an exotoxin which acts on the nervous system in several ways. It excites the local motor nerves producing muscular spasm in the neighbourhood of the injury. This is the earliest effect. The toxin may then reach the central nervous system, where it causes a stiffness of the muscles of the face, producing 'trismus' or 'lockjaw'. It excites the motor nerves of muscles in various parts of the body, producing muscular spasms. These come on in paroxysms which may be very severe. In the most serious cases, virtually all the muscles of the body may be involved, producing the hyperextended condition known as 'opisthotonus'.

Tetanus is always a serious and a very painful disease. The mildest cases have to be treated with great care, in silence and in a darkened room, since the extent to which toxin may reach the central nervous system cannot be predicted and any disturbance may bring on a spasm.

Once toxin has reached the central nervous system, its action on the motor nerves may be prevented by curariform drugs which have been used with success in the treatment of tetanus. General anaesthetics may also reduce the excitability of the patient. When paroxysms are severe there is a danger of the trachea being blocked by mucus, and tracheotomy may be necessary.

Laboratory Diagnosis

Examination of swabs from the wound:
1. Microscopy of stained smears.
2. Culture.

Treatment

Large doses of antitoxin intravenously, with penicillin or tetracyclines. Treatment of spasms and respiratory failure by appropriate methods.

Prevention

The prevention of tetanus is an important problem with which doctors in hospitals and in general practice are frequently faced.

Children should be actively immunised with toxoid at an early age. If they at any time afterwards receive an injury which appears to carry a danger of tetanus, their immunity can be boosted with another dose of toxoid. All servicemen are actively immunised in this way.

However, most people are unfortunately not so immunised at present. A difficult problem for the general practitioner, or for casualty doctors in hospitals, is the prophylactic treatment of an unimmunised, wounded person. Theoretically it should be possible to prevent tetanus in every case of tetanus-prone injury by giving a dose of antitoxin, and for many years this was the accepted form of treatment. However, it is unsatisfactory for two reasons. The first is that tetanus antitoxin is not a safe drug. It is made usually from horses' serum to which many people are allergic, and may give rise to troublesome reactions, particularly in patients with a history of allergy, such as asthmatics or children or adults with eczema. Occasionally these reactions are fatal. Patients should never be given a dose of tetanus antitoxin without first having a small injection of a test dose subcutaneously, to see if they have any general reaction. Even if they do not, they should not be given the full dose without being kept under observation for at least 20 minutes.

Secondly, the effect of antitoxin given in this way may not last for very long. At best, the protection will last for several weeks. However, there are cases in which it may last only for a few days. This happens in people who have previously been 'sensitised' by doses of horse serum, for previous protection either against tetanus or possibly diphtheria. An infected wound will often harbour tetanus bacilli and be dangerous for longer than this.

If the wound is seen by a doctor soon after it occurs, surgical treatment should be performed and should include adequate excision. In practice, however, this is often not possible. The wound may be in a part full of vital structures, such as the hand, or it may be too small for excision to be practicable. Sometimes tetanus occurs in patients whose wound was so small and apparently trivial that they were not aware of a wound at all.

Because of the difficulties and dangers of prophylactic horse-serum antitoxin, many people think today that this substance should be dropped altogether, and reliance be placed on antibiotics such as penicillin or tetracycline, with surgical excision when possible, for the prevention of tetanus.

A recent development with promise for the future is the introduction of antitoxin made from human serum. Unlike horse serum, this does not give rise to allergic reactions. It is expensive, but it is a practical and safe alternative to horse antitoxin.

If all infants were actively immunised with toxoid, the problem of prophylactic antitoxin would never arise.

The differences between Active Immunisation (toxoid) and Passive Immunisation (antitoxin) are discussed more fully in Chapter 10.

Botulism

Botulism is a very rare but very serious form of food poisoning caused by *Clostridium botulinum*. The organism forms a toxin which is swallowed in the food and is responsible for the disease. The patient develops paralysis of the peripheral nerves and death may occur when the central nervous system is affected. If the disease is diagnosed in time, the only effective treatment is antitoxin.

Spirochaetal Infections

Syphilis

The most serious of the venereal diseases is *Syphilis*. This is due to a spirochaete called *Treponema pallidum*. Syphilis is serious because long after the initial infection the organism may spread in the bloodstream and produce chronic and fatal disease of the blood vessels, liver, heart or

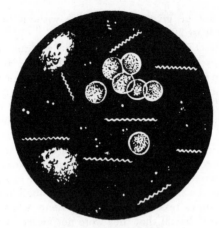

Fig. 27. Treponema pallidum

nervous system. It may cause a fatal aneurysm, or paralysis, or brain damage forty years after the sexual contact which produced infection. It may be transmitted by a mother to her children, producing congenital syphilis. This may take the form of physical deformity, or heart disease, or nervous disease from which the child may never fully recover.

The infection may be transmitted to or from men or women and usually enters the new host either via the genital organs or via the mouth. About a fortnight after implantation it causes a hard, painless nodule or *Chancre*. At this stage the local lymph nodes may be swollen but are painless. This is called the **primary stage**, and disappears after a few weeks. The microbe travels all over the body via the blood-stream, and after a few more weeks the **secondary stage** begins. This takes the form of a generalised infection with fever, a copper-red rash, generalised painless enlargement of the lymph nodes, malaise, headaches, and sore throat. At this stage, shallow ulcers may appear on the tongue or the mucous membrane of the mouth, and raised patches called **condylomas** in moist areas such as the perineum. All these lesions are highly infective.

In the absence of treatment, the secondary stage usually subsides after a few weeks. Months or years afterwards the **tertiary stage** begins, with lesions in almost any part of the body which take the form of fibrous nodules or **gummas**. Finally the late manifestations already mentioned may occur.

Laboratory Diagnosis

1. Microscopy.
During the **primary stage** it may be possible to demonstrate the treponema microscopically in scrapings from the chancre using a special technique called dark ground illumination.
2. Serological tests.

A few weeks after the infection, before the onset of the second stage, the blood tests become positive. A widely used test is the Wassermann reaction, which is a complement fixation test. In recent years, several other reliable tests have come into use in Great Britain, such as the Treponema pallidum immobilisation (TPI) and haemagglutination (HA) tests. In syphilis of the central nervous system the cerebrospinal fluid may give positive results.

Between 5 and 10ml of blood in a plain tube is needed for the serological tests for syphilis. They are laborious tests which take up much time, so they are usually done in batches once or twice a week.

Prevention and Treatment

Syphilis, like gonorrhoea, is spread by sexual promiscuity. The most important preventive measure is the prevention of promiscuity.

In the first few days after the infection the disease may be prevented by antibiotics. Penicillin, to which the organism is very sensitive, is used as a rule. The treatment remains fairly simple until the second stage of the disease after which it becomes increasingly difficult. In the tertiary, or late stages, several courses of treatment each lasting about a fortnight may be necessary and may need to be supplemented with arsenical drugs or bismuth. Congenital syphilis may be prevented by treatment of the mother during pregnancy.

Yaws is an endemic disease similar to syphilis which is found in Africa. It is caused by *Treponema pertenue*, and is spread by any kind of contact, not necessarily sexual.

Leptospirosis—Weil's Disease

Weil's disease, or spirochaetal jaundice, is due to an organism called *Leptospira icterohaemorrhagica*. This infection is spread in the urine of rats and occurs in people who are in contact with rats. It therefore occurs in sewage workers, dwellers in damp basements, and people who fall into, or bathe in canals. It used to be a common disease in the fishworkers of Dundee and Aberdeen who processed fresh fish in large rat-infested sheds by the waterside. There are rare varieties of Weil's disease spread by other animals, one of them by dogs.

Weil's disease takes the form of an acute infection of the liver with jaundice; the kidneys may also be affected.

Laboratory Diagnosis

Microscopy and culture of organisms from the blood or urine. Examination of serum for antibodies.

Antibiotic treatment

Penicillin or tetracyclines.

Vincent's Angina

This is a mild but unpleasant infection of the mucous membrane of the mouth and pharynx. It is due to a spirochaete which looks like the syphilis organism but is much less serious in its effects. This is called *Borrelia vincenti*.

Laboratory Diagnosis

Microscopy of smears from the mouth.

Antibiotic treatment

Penicillin.

Relapsing Fever

This is an endemic disease in many parts of the world, chiefly Eastern Europe, Central Asia, India, Africa, and Central and South America. It is due to various species of spirochaete (*Borrelia*), and is spread by the bites of ticks and lice.

Laboratory Diagnosis

1. Microscopy of stained blood smear.
2. Serological tests.

Antibiotic treatment

Penicillin or tetracyclines.

CHAPTER 6

THE MAIN TYPES OF INFECTIVE ILLNESS—
VIRUS INFECTIONS

Some of the commonest infectious diseases in the world are virus diseases. Certainly in Great Britain, *colds*, which are virus infections, are by far the commonest illnesses.

In this chapter, virus infections are dealt with under the following headings, which are based not on the classification of viruses, but on convenient clinical groupings:

1. Virus diseases with a prominent skin rash.
2. Virus infections of the respiratory tract.
3. Virus infections of the nervous system.
4. Other virus infections and rickettsial infections.

1. Virus Diseases with a Prominent Skin Rash

The common fevers associated with a rash, which used to be called the Exanthems, are nearly all virus diseases. However, the effects of these diseases are by no means confined to the skin, and in many cases, the virus enters the body through the respiratory tract. In most of these diseases there is a phase, before the rash appears, in which the virus circulates in the blood-stream and can be recovered from the blood.

Measles

This is due to a virus which was isolated a few years ago. Infection takes place by droplets through the respiratory tract. Most people suffer an attack of measles in childhood, and enjoy immunity for the rest of their lives. The disease is extremely infectious. It starts as a catarrhal respiratory infection with fever, and in a few days the rash 'breaks out'.

Incubation period

Usually 10 days to the onset of fever, 14 days to the onset of the rash. This may be longer if gamma globulin has been administered.

Laboratory Diagnosis

1. Isolation of the virus from nasopharynx, blood, or urine.
2. Detection of antibodies in serum.

Treatment

No specific treatment.

Prevention

1. Isolation of cases and contacts.
2. Immunisation.

In Great Britain, a vaccine containing attenuated virus is used for protection against measles. It is also possible to protect immunised children exposed to the disease, at least for a time, by means of immuno-globulin **(IgG)**. This is a form of passive immunisation (see Chapter 10).

If the administration of IgG is delayed for a few days after contact, modified measles may result. This is a mild form of the disease which yet gives full immunity against further attacks.

Rubella (German Measles)

This is a trivial disease of childhood, of which a single attack usually brings life-long immunity. In adult life the disease may be quite unpleasant, though it is usually mild. Until the early 1940s, rubella was regarded as of little importance. At that time, however, it was discovered that an attack of rubella in expectant mothers early in pregnancy might give rise to serious congenital defects in their infants. This discovery was made in Australia, where after a severe epidemic of rubella it was noticed than an unusually large number of children were born with congenital blindness, or deafness, or both. This led to a world-wide study of the effects of rubella in early pregnancy. It is now known that an attack of rubella in the second and third months of pregnancy carries an appreciable risk to the infant, something like one chance in four or five, of its being born with a serious defect. This may be blindness, deafness, heart disease, malformation of the brain, or a combination of these.

The realisation of this risk brings up the problem of prevention, which is twofold: first, how can disease be prevented in the infant of an infected expectant mother? Secondly, are there any general measures to prevent this type of congenital disease?

So far as the first problem is concerned, there is virtually no risk in the case of a mother who has a clear history of rubella in the past. The problem is, however, a frequent one in mothers who have never had rubella, or who are uncertain whether they have had the disease or not. The only preventive measure which is at all likely to be effective is to give them a dose of IgG (see Chapter 10). This may well prevent the onset of infection, if it is given within eight days of exposure.

The answer to the second question is simple. All girls should contract rubella before they reach child-bearing age. This is the surest way to prevent congenital disease due to this cause. Infection in little girls should be welcomed, not avoided, with one proviso — that their mothers have had rubella and are not in the early stages of pregnancy at the time. For the little girl may, of course, infect her pregnant mother.

If it is suspected that a pregnant woman has contracted rubella, this can be confirmed or disproved by testing her blood for the presence of antibodies. A negative result rules out infection.

Immunisation with vaccines is now widely performed.

Incubation period — 14 to 21 days.

Laboratory diagnosis — Same tests as in measles.

Treatment — None specific.

Prevention — See above.

Chickenpox (Varicella)

This is another acute exanthem of childhood, usually, but not always, mild. It is caused by the same virus as **Herpes zoster**, a disease with a localised rash which occurs in infected contacts of chickenpox who have had that disease many years before, and so have some immunity, but not enough to prevent infection entirely. Contacts of cases of either chickenpox or herpes zoster may themselves contract either disease, according to their state of immunity. Those with some immunity from past infection may develop herpes zoster, while those with no immunity are likely to develop chickenpox.

Incubation period — Chickenpox: 12 to 16 days. Zoster: 7 to 14 days.

Laboratory diagnosis — Similar to Smallpox.

Treatment — None specific.

Prevention — Avoidance of contact.

Herpes zoster is not to be confused with **Herpes simplex**. This is a disease caused by a virus which many people 'carry' in their facial nerves in the latent state. When they are 'run down' or suffering from some other infection they may develop a 'cold sore' on the face near the mouth — **Herpes labialis**.

Gingivostomatitis — numberous small blisters inside the mouth — is a common form of herpes simplex infection seen in small children.

Herpetic whitlow is a painful infection of the finger which may occur in nurses and others in contact with patients who carry the Herpes virus.

Smallpox (Variola)

This is one of the most serious of virus diseases. The virus enters the body through the mucous membrane of the upper respiratory tract; it is transmitted either by direct contact from an infected case, by droplet infection or from handling something which has been very recently handled by a patient with smallpox.

Incubation period

10 to 14 days.

Laboratory Diagnosis

1. In the pre-eruptive stage (after the start of fever, but before the rash appears): Isolation of virus from the blood.
2. After rash has appeared:
   (a) Microscopy of fluid from pox, to detect virus particles;
   (b) Culture of virus from pox on chick embryos in eggs;
   (c) Testing pox fluid with antiserum to detect virus.
3. After one week of illness: Detection of antibody in serum.

Treatment

No specific treatment at time of writing. However, there is much research in progress on producing suitable drugs.

Prevention

1. Isolation of cases and avoidance of contacts.
2. Vaccination.

The only sure way of preventing smallpox is by vaccination. This means the introduction into the skin of a virus related to the smallpox or variola virus which is called vaccinia. Vaccination is followed by what is, in effect, a mild disease, consisting usually of a small blister and some enlargement of the regional lymph nodes; there may also be some general symptoms, especially in people who have not been vaccinated before. However, vaccination confers a long-lasting immunity to smallpox owing to the fact that the viruses of the two diseases, vaccinia and smallpox, are closely related. It also confers immunity to itself, which means that after vaccination people cannot be successfully revaccinated for some time, a year or more, as they are immune.

The process of vaccination was invented by an English country doctor named Edward Jenner, who practised in Gloucestershire towards the end of the eighteenth century. During a serious epidemic of smallpox, Jenner noticed that milkmaids who had previously suffered from cowpox were immune. Cowpox is a mild disease of cattle which milkmaids might contract by contact with the udders of infected cows; in humans it takes the form of a series of blisters in the skin rather like vaccinia. Jenner conceived the idea of immunising large numbers of people against smallpox by giving them cowpox infection deliberately; this was the original process of vaccination. However, the modern vaccinia vaccines are slightly different from cowpox.

In recent years, an international campaign has almost succeeded in eliminating smallpox. At the time of writing there are very few places in the world where the disease is still to be found. This is an outstanding example of successful international co-operation.

Some countries may require visitors to be vaccinated.

After a primary vaccination, a papule appears in about four days. This becomes vesicular by the seventh day. It then subsides, leaving a crusted dry lesion in about twelve days. After three weeks it has almost disappeared.

Complications of vaccination

The local lesion may be quite large, there may be tenderness and enlargement of the local lymph nodes, and the patient may suffer malaise and headache.

The serious complications of vaccination are rare and are meningo-encephalitis and generalised vaccinia, in which the reaction, instead of consisting of a single blister, takes the form of a series of vesicles all over the body.

These reactions denote the absence of immunity to vaccinia. They may be fatal.

2. Virus Diseases chiefly affecting the Respiratory Tract: The Common Cold

For years, much research has been done on this troublesome disease, which is the commonest of all virus diseases, and which causes millions of days of sickness annually. It is now known that colds are not caused by a single virus, but by any of a large number of viruses.

This means that there are formidable technical difficulties to be overcome before an effective vaccine is produced. It would have to contain many different strains of each of these viruses in sufficient concentration to produce immunity.

The various vaccines against the common cold which are already in use are non-specific in their action. Some of these provide antibodies against microbes which cause respiratory complications of colds, such as the bacterium *Haemophilus influenzae*. Others owe their effectiveness, if any, to morale-boosting rather than to any objective stimulation of immunity.

Influenza

There are known to be three types of influenza virus, called A, B, and C. There are many strains of each type; indeed, new strains are continually arising by mutation and each new epidemic is usually caused by a strain slightly different from those of previous epidemics. Most epidemics in this country are caused by strains of either A or B viruses. Influenza epidemics are rarely confined to a single country; usually they spread all over the world from the area in which they first arise. It is thus often possible to predict an epidemic of influenza; when a new strain crops up anywhere in the world it is likely to spread to other parts. There is a World Influenza Centre in London where strains from all over the world are collected so that such predictions may be made. Thus, a few years ago, a European outbreak was successfully predicted because of the occurrence of a new strain, the 'Asiatic virus', in Malaya.

The importance of this is that it is now possible to prepare in advance large amounts of virus of the predicted epidemic strain in order to prepare vaccines for immunisation purposes. A widespread immunisation campaign could therefore cut short an outbreak.

Commercial vaccines, containing mixtures of past epidemic strains, are already much used. While they are not likely to be so effective in preventing influenza as a vaccine made against the actual epidemic strain, none the less they do seem to have some value. However, none of these vaccines will protect against colds, only against influenza.

Before the discovery of the virus in the 1930s it was thought that influenza was due to a bacterium, *Haemophilus influenzae* (see page 45). It is now known that this microbe may cause a secondary pheumonia in cases of influenza; it may also cause meningitis, particularly in children.

Laboratory Diagnosis

In colds and influenza is rarely practical, but the following are possible methods:
1. Isolation of virus from nasal washings.
2. Detection of antibodies in serum.

Treatment

No specific treatment.

Prevention

1. Avoidance of contact.
2. Vaccination — see above.

Virus Pneumonia

There are many viruses which cause 'virus pneumonia', or 'primary atypical pneumonia'. The influenza viruses themselves may do this; so may

Respiratory Syncitial (RS) virus which causes severe pneumonia in infants. *Rickettsia burneti* causes a type of pneumonia called Q fever. Psittacosis, or 'parrot fever', is a pneumonia of birds which may attack human beings, usually after contact with infected parrots or other birds. It is due to a virus.

Laboratory Diagnosis

1. Isolation of virus from blood and urine.
2. Detection of antibodies in serum.

Treatment

In Q fever – Tetracyclines and chloramphenicol.

Prevention

Avoidance of contact.
  No immunisation possible.

Mumps

Mumps is caused by a type of virus called a **myxovirus** which usually enters the body via inhaled droplets. The disease takes the form of a painful enlargement of one or more of the salivary glands, accompanied by fever. Occasionally, the virus may attack the testes or ovaries, causing orchitis or oophoritis, or it may cause pancreatitis or encephalitis.

Incubation period

17 to 21 days.

Laboratory Diagnosis

Similar to those for influenza.

Treatment

No specific treatment. Antibiotics have no effect.

Prevention

Avoidance of contact with cases, who are infectious from about 24 hours before the onset of swelling until the time that the swelling subsides.
  Gamma globulin may prevent attacks in contacts.
  Vaccination.

Trachoma and Inclusion Conjunctivitis

The **trachoma** agent, now called 'chlamydia', is the cause of a very common form of conjunctivitis. The acute disease often leads to permanent scarring which is one of the chief causes of blindness throughout the Far and Middle East and North Africa. As many as four hundred million people are thought to be affected throughout the world.

The disease is spread by contact of any infected objects such as fingers and clothing with the eyes. It may also be transmitted from the mother to her child, and may be spread by flies.

Inclusion Conjunctivitis is a mild epidemic disease caused by the same chlamydia.

Laboratory Diagnosis

Scrapings from the conjunctiva should be examined thus:
1. Microscopy for inclusion bodies.
2. Culture of virus.

Treatment

Tetracyclines, chloramphenicol, sulphonamides.

Prevention

Improved sanitation.

It is possible that a vaccine will soon be available, but this is not yet the case.

Enterovirus Infections

The enteroviruses are viruses which enter the body through the alimentary tract, after being swallowed or inhaled into the mouth or pharynx. They multiply in the tonsils or the Peyer's patches of the small intestine and then travel via the blood stream and throughout the body.

Different members of the group cause disease in different organs, such as the central nervous system, the muscles, and the heart. Some of them are responsible for colds. On the other hand, infection by these viruses is very often subclinical; that is to say, they may not cause any disease at all.

There are many enteroviruses, and their classification is still the subject of much research and discussion. They are very small, among the smallest of all viruses. They are usually cultured on tissue cultures of human or monkey cells.

Enteroviruses fall into three main groups:
1. The Polioviruses.
2. The Coxsackie viruses.
3. The ECHO viruses.

Both the Coxsackie and ECHO groups may cause disease varying from head colds to fever with pain in the chest and aseptic meningitis. On the whole these illnesses are benign, that is to say, they clear up without any serious sequels.

Poliomyelitis is much more serious as it may lead to permanent paralysis.

Laboratory Diagnosis of Coxsackie and Echo infections:

1. Isolation of virus from the faeces.
2. Demonstration of antibodies in the serum.

Treatment

No specific treatment.

Poliomyelitis and Polioencephalitis

There are three distinct types of poliovirus; immunity against one does not confer immunity against any of the others. There are several strains of each type, some of which are virulent and some are not. Polioviruses live in the alimentary tract of cases of the disease or of carriers. The most important method of spread is by the faeces; indeed, examination of the sewage of any locality for poliovirus is used as a means of detecting carriers. Poliomyelitis may also be spread by droplet infection from the mouth.

Once it infects the alimentary tract of a new case, the virus crosses the mucous membrane and enters the blood stream. It may cause no clinical disease at all, or a full-blown attack of paralytic poliomyelitis, or any grade of disease in between these two extremes. What actually occurs depends on the two decisive factors, the virulence of the organism and the resistance of the host.

In a typical case of poliomyelitis, the illness begins with a heavy cold, possibly accompanied by a headache. This is the catarrhal stage and the disease may get no further. Then a rise of temperature may occur, with intense pains in one or more limbs; after a few hours, paralysis may start and the patient finds difficulty in moving a limb, or has some weakness in it. This paralysis occurs when the virus has attacked the anterior horn cells of the motor nerves in the spinal cord.

If the patient is given complete rest at this stage, recovery usually occurs, and is complete after a few days. However, the course of an attack of poliomyelitis is unpredictable in the early stages. Paralysis may spread rapidly, involving the respiratory muscles so that the patient cannot breathe for himself but has to be given some mechanical help from a respirator. The inflammation of the central nervous system may spread up into the brain, producing coma; this is **polioencephalitis**.

It is known that exertion or mechanical damage is likely to make the disease worse, and rest improves the outlook. So as soon as poliomyelitis is suspected, the patient should be put to bed and kept there. If any limb is particularly painful, it should be rested. As soon as possible, the patient should be admitted to a fever hospital where there are both the respiratory apparatus for dealing with cases of respiratory poliomyelitis and nurses skilled in the special treatment required. Respiratory paralysis may occur very rapidly, and if the patient happens to be in a place where immediate help is not forthcoming, serious and permanent paralysis, or even death may result.

As is well known, poliomyelitis may lead to irreparable damage of the nerve cells and to lasting paralysis. After the disease has subsided, however even if some muscles are permanently damaged, neighbouring muscles take over their function to a large extent, and may produce almost complete functional recovery. Most cases of paralytic poliomyelitis recover completely. But there are a minority who remain disabled, and sometimes seriously, for the rest of their lives. A still smaller number die in the acute stage of the illness. The extent of the recovery depends to a large extent on the efforts which the patient himself makes, and a cheerful optimistic outlook is very helpful.

Laboratory Diagnosis

No specific tests are of practical value in the early stages, and in practice the diagnosis is usually made on clinical grounds. It can be proved however, by:
1. Isolation of the virus from the stools.
2. Detection of antibodies in serum.

Treatment

No specific antibiotic treatment. The treatment of poliomyelitis is outside the scope of this book.

Prevention

There are two sides to this:
1. **The prevention of the spread of poliovirus**. As the virus is usually spread by faecal contamination, this is a matter of food hygiene and is the same as the prevention of typhoid, salmonella and dysentery infections.
2. **Immunisation**. Poliomyelitis can be prevented by immunisation, and every child should be immunised. There are two different kinds of vaccine available, both of which are effective. Attenuated (live) vaccine consists of a mixture of the three types of poliovirus in an attenuated, or weakened, state. In this form it may multiply in the gut producing immunity, but cannot invade the cells of the central nervous system. It may be administered on a lump of sugar or in a drink; three doses at monthly intervals should be given. Inactivated (killed) vaccine has to be given by injection. It has the advantage that it can be combined with other vaccines

such as diphtheria, whooping cough and tetanus, in a single series of injections.

It is not yet known for how long poliomyelitis immunisation remains effective. However, since the introduction of immunisation, the incidence of poliomyelitis has fallen throughout the world very markedly.

Cases of paralytic poliomyelitis have been shown to follow intense exertion, for instance, competitive athletics, during epidemics. They have also followed other kinds of trauma. Sometimes children develop paralytic poliomyelitis within a few days of an injection, such as diphtheria immunisation. In such cases, the paralysed limb is always the one in which the injection has been made. It is thought that the injection 'activates' the virus in some way, causing it to attack the anterior horn cells serving the injected limb. Patients have developed poliomyelitis soon after tonsillectomy operations. Possibly, the operation causes a breach in the mucous membrane of the pharynx through which the virus can get into the blood stream or reach the central nervous system. During outbreaks of poliomyelitis, it is advisable to reduce the number of tonsillectomy operations to a minimum, and to perform as few injections as possible.

Other Virus Diseases of the Central Nervous System

In addition to poliomyelitis, there are numerous other virus diseases of the central nervous system. Many different viruses cause meningitis; one variety is 'benign aseptic meningitis', so-called because the patient nearly always recovers completely, and there is no paralysis. Other viruses which cause this disease include the ECHO viruses, the LCM viruses which cause lymphocytic choriomeningitis and the Coxsackie viruses. The latter may also cause 'Bornholm disease', an acute illness with fever and intense muscular pains rather like a fibrositis.

Encephalitis

There are many varieties of virus **encephalitis**. Some of the causes, such as poliovirus, mumps, and smallpox virus, have already been mentioned. The commonest types of virus encephalitis occur in the tropics and are carried by arthropods such as mosquitoes, mites or ticks. Encephalitis is often mild. Sometimes, however, it is an acute and serious disease which may end fatally within a few days. Vaccination with some virus vaccines, such as smallpox, may give rise to encephalitis as a complication.

Laboratory Diagnosis

Lumbar puncture shows increase in lymphocytes.
   Isolation of virus from the stool.
   Demonstration of antibodies in serum.

Treatment

No specific treatment.

Prevention

No specific measures known.

Rabies

This is a very serious disease which occurs after the bite of an infected dog, wolf, fox, bat and some other animals. The disease takes the form of an acute encephalitis, in which any disturbance, such as the sound of running water, may cause acute distress. The disease is usually fatal.

Laboratory Diagnosis

Infected animals can be detected for certain only when they are dead. Section of the brain reveals the specific inclusion bodies or 'Negri bodies' in the nerve cells.

Incubation period

From two weeks to several months.

Treatment

No specific treatment.

Prevention

1. Control of infected animals.

Rabies can be prevented only by the rigid control of dogs and other animals which carry the infection. In Great Britain, freedom from rabies has been maintained by the strict quarantine of all imported animals.

At the time of writing, there is serious danger that rabies may be imported from the European Continent. If this happens, it may be impossible to prevent the spread of the disease in this country.

2. Vaccination of bitten people.

If a person is bitten by an animal suspected to be infected, the disease can often be prevented by a course of injections of Pasteur's vaccine, which consists of extracts of the dried spinal cord of affected animals. It is a long and painful course of injections, but none the less, it is better than an attack of the disease.

Virus Hepatitis

There are three main varieties of virus hepatitis. One is **infective hepatitis** or hepatitis A. This is due to a virus found in the alimentary tract of cases, so that the disease may spread by faecal contamination. It may also spread by droplet infection.

Incubation period — 15-40 days.

Laboratory Diagnosis — No specific tests.

Prevention

General hygienic measures as for typhoid, salmonella and dysentery infections.

Immunisation with human immunoglobulin gives short term protection and is recommended for travellers to countries where hepatitis is endemic.

Hepatitis B, serum hepatitis, syringe-transmitted jaundice, Australia antigen hepatitis, homologous serum jaundice. This may be spread by contact with infected blood or blood products, or by injections in which infected syringes or needles are used. The incubation period of this disease is very long, up to six months. This means that future sufferers from the disease may carry the organism in their blood stream for up to six months without being suspected of being carriers.

Incubation period — 45 days to 6 months.

Laboratory Diagnosis — Blood test for the detection of the hepatitis B antigen.

Treatment — None specific.

Prevention

General hygienic measures in the handling of blood and blood products. A sterile syringe and needle should be used for *every* injection and vene-puncture.

It is now known that many people are carriers of both the above types of hepatitis virus, and the blood, faeces, and urine of such carriers may be infective. Outbreaks of hepatitis frequently occur in renal dialysis units among both patients and staff. Cases may also occur among the staff of chemical pathology, haematology, and immunology laboratories, indeed of any laboratories in which the work involves contact with blood specimens.

There are several laboratory tests for the presence of Australia antigen (virus), or the antibody to it, in the serum of suspected cases or carriers. At the time of writing it is not agreed which are the best tests for routine use.

A third type of virus hepatitis is **Yellow Fever**, which occurs in tropical Africa and Central America. The virus is carried by the bite of a mosquito, *Aedes aegypti*. The disease starts with a fever, headache, and backache, which is soon followed by nausea and vomiting. There may be gastric haemorrhage, followed by vomit containing altered blood. In severe cases, the blood pressure falls, the heart rate slows, and the kidneys also are affected; such cases are often fatal. In non-fatal cases, recovery is usually complete.

Incubation period

3 to 6 days.

Laboratory Diagnosis

1. Isolation of virus from the blood.
2. Detection of antibodies in serum.

Treatment

None specific.

Prevention

1. The control of mosquitoes.
2. Immunisation.

Everyone visiting the 'yellow fever' belt of Africa should be immunised before making the journey. A single injection gives protection for ten years.

Rickettsial Infections

The *Rickettsias* are the largest known viruses, though some workers do not regard them as viruses at all. They are responsible for various kinds of **typhus**, and also for Q fever which was mentioned on page 26. Typhus is a serious systemic fever: the disease is often fatal unless antibiotics are used.

In all kinds of typhus, the rickettsias reach human beings by way of an arthropod host — a louse, flea, mite or tick.

Epidemic typhus, which is louse-borne, occurs in overcrowded communities with low standards of living. It has always been common in Eastern Europe, especially during and after the two world wars.

The disease is liable to spread through whole villages as lice spread from one person to another. Blankets, bedding and tents may all be infected in any typhus-ridden community. The control of typhus depends on the de-lousing of the community and their bedding. Thanks to modern insecticides such as DDT and Gammexane, this no longer is as difficult as it was, but it can still be a formidable undertaking.

Endemic typhus affects rats as well as human beings, and is carried from rats to humans by fleas. The disease occurs all over the world in cities with infected rat populations. The control of the disease depends on the hunting and destruction of infected rats and on the control of human infestation by fleas.

A **mite-borne** type of typhus occurs in the Far East and Japan; this is called **Scrub Typhus**. As in endemic typhus, the main reservoir is rats.

Tick-borne typhus occurs in various parts of the world and is named after the location; thus there are Rocky Mountain Spotted Fever, Mediterranean Fever, Siberian Typhus, North Queensland Typhus and so on.

Laboratory Diagnosis

1. Isolation of rickettsias from blood.
2. Demonstration of antibodies in serum.

Treatment

Chloramphenicol or tetracyclines.

Prevention

(a) Breaking the chain of infection:
   Epidemic typhus—delousing with DDT.
   Endemic typhus—control of fleas. Eradication of rats. Rat-proofing buildings.
   Scrub-typhus and tick-typhus—clearing sites where rats and mites live.
(b) Vaccination, using vaccines grown on chick embryos in eggs.

Glandular Fever (Infectious mononucleosis)

This is almost certainly a virus infection due to an organism called the Epstein-Barr virus. It is infectious and is spread by such contact as 'deep kissing' (it has been called the 'kissing disease').

Laboratory Diagnosis

1. Examination of white blood cells—abnormal mononuclear cells are seen in the blood.
2. Detection of abnormal antibodies in serum (Paul-Bunnell test).

CHAPTER 7

THE MAIN TYPES OF INFECTIVE ILLNESS —
PATHOGENIC FUNGI

Pathogenic fungi are among the commonest causes of infection. Fungal infections are usually mild and superficial, though deep-seated infections also occur which may be extremely serious.

The Dermatophytes

The dermatophytes are a group of fungi which cause ringworm, athlete's foot, and similar infections of the skin. Many of these can live on keratin, and attack the hairs of the scalp. They may also live in fingernails and toenails. In addition to hairy skin or that around the nails, skin which is often moist is also liable to be attacked by fungi. This means the skin of flexures such as those between the legs, in the axillae, under the breasts of a woman, and between the toes.

Dermatophyte infections are extremely common and they are often chronic and may go on for years. Or they may recur again and again after apparent cure. Usually they do not cause much disability, but they frequently give rise to troublesome itching and may cause deformity, particularly of the fingernails and toenails. They may also become secondarily infected and give rise to serious illness in this way.

Ringworm of the scalp and skin often causes epidemics in communities such as schools and military units. Athlete's foot is commonly endemic in swimming baths and changing rooms.

Laboratory Diagnosis

Examination of scrapings or scales or hairs by **microscopy** and **culture**. Fresh material should be teased out in 10% caustic soda or potash, and looked at under the microscope, when the fungus can easily be seen as slender branching filaments among the cells. This examination is often made in the out-patient's clinic.

Culture on special media such as Sabouraud's media may take two or three weeks to show a growth. The different fungi concerned have different cultural appearances, but most show a fluffy mould-like growth. Some, such as *Trichophyton rubrum* which is red, produce a characteristic pigment.

Treatment

Local, with antifungal ointments or paints.

General — Griseofulvin, an antibiotic, is taken by mouth for long periods and usually cures even the most persistent dermatophyte infections such as that due to *Trichophyton rubrum*, which is perhaps the most troublesome of all this group of organisms.

Prevention

General hygienic measures as follows: Keep socks and underclothes of infected cases away from those of other people. Liberal use of fungicidal dusting powders, ointments, and creams.

Prevention of contact with known cases.

Frequent disinfection of the floors of swimming baths, changing rooms, etc.

Candida albicans

The thrush fungus (formerly called 'Monilia')

This is a yeast-like fungus which is the cause of thrush, a mild disease of the mouth affecting people of all ages, especially newborn infants. Oral thrush of infants may occur as an epidemic in nurseries and be spread by infected feeding bottles or teats. In adults, thrush commonly occurs in the vagina, particularly during pregnancy. Mothers with vaginal thrush may give the disease to their infants. Vaginal thrush may be a chronic infection; it gives rise to an itchy discharge which may be very troublesome. *Candida albicans* is the commonest cause of vaginal discharge; the other common cause is the flagellate protozoon *Trichomonas vaginalis*.

Candida albicans may also cause disease of the skin, particularly of the flexures of the body. The fingernails may be affected in housewives and other occupational groups, such as barmen and fishmongers, whose hands are frequently wettened. Rarely, *Candida albicans* may cause disease of the lungs or other parts of the body.

Laboratory Diagnosis

Microscopy and **culture** of fresh material.

Treatment

Nystatin, by local application.

Prevention

In newborn infants: Sterilisation of feeding bottles and teats. Scrupulous attention to general nursery hygiene (see page 92), where cross-infection is liable to occur. Mothers with vaginal thrush should be particularly careful about washing their hands before handling or feeding their babies.

Vaginal thrush: Personal hygiene.

Skin and fingernails: Keep flexures dry and hands as dry as possible.

The Aspergilli

The Aspergilli are a widespread group of fungi; their spores are often present in dust and are found in the air. *Aspergillus niger* is frequently found in superficial cavities such as the external ear. *Aspergillus fumigatus* causes a lung disease called **aspergilloma**. This starts as a mass of debris in a cavity of a diseased lung, or in a patch of bronchiectasis; it becomes colonised with aspergillus spores inhaled from the air. Aspergillomas may be quite large and may persist for years; the only effective treatment is surgical removal.

Actinomycosis

This is a rare disease caused by a fungus called *Actinomyces israeli*. The disease is a chronic inflammation, often with the formation of persistent and troublesome sinuses; the jaw, the lungs, the liver or the gut may be affected.

The organisms are often found in the mouth of healthy people. Actinomycosis of the jaw has occasionally followed extraction of a tooth. Even more rarely, a human bite has been followed by actinomycosis at the site of the bite.

There is a copious discharge of pus from the lesions, and the pus contains small 'sulphur granules'; these, when squashed, stained, and examined under the microscope, consist of a central mass of fine filaments of actinomyces, surrounded by lighter-staining tissue debris.

Laboratory Diagnosis

Microscopy and culture of pus from a suspected case.

Treatment

Penicillin.

Prevention

None.

Other Pathogenic Fungi

There are many other types of deep-seated fungal infection which are all uncommon. Some, such as the *Nocardias*, cause chronic inflammatory disease with sinus formation, resembling actinomycosis. Others, such as *Histoplasma* and *Coccidioides*, cause a chronic infection of the chest. *Blastomycosis* is often associated with granulomatous skin lesions. *Cryptococcus neoformans* may cause serious infection anywhere in the body, and cryptococcal meningitis is usually fatal.

CHAPTER 8

MICROBIOLOGY IN DAY-TO-DAY PATIENT CARE

The importance of microbiology in the care of patients cannot be over-emphasised. Every contact with the patient brings with it the possibility of infection and raises the problem of its avoidance.

Florence Nightingale wrote in 1863: 'It may seem a strange principle to enunciate as the very first requirement in a hospital that it should do the sick no harm. It is quite necessary, nevertheless, to lay down such a principle'.

Today, over a hundred years later, it is still necessary. Thoughtless or careless actions by the nurse or other people looking after patients may cause an unnecessary and avoidable infection which may add several days, or weeks, to the patient's stay in hospital, or have more serious and even fatal effects. This kind of thing happens quite frequently. Most often it is not noticed at the time. There are many hospitals in which patients are overcrowded, and cross-infection of one patient by another is difficult to avoid. None the less, it *can* be avoided by proper care and attention on the part of the staff.

While nurses probably play the largest role in the avoidance of hospital infection, they are not the only people concerned. The behaviour of doctors is equally important. Domestic staff and porters also play a large part. A careless action on the part of anyone in a surgical ward or operating theatre may start an outbreak of infection. Radiologists, physiotherapists, occupational therapists, all who come into contact with patients, should have some knowledge of the cause and prevention of hospital infections. Even those whose contact with patients is only indirect, such as staff of the central sterile supply departments, catering staff, and administrative staff, may by their actions cause or prevent outbreaks of infection.

It is impossible to look after sick people without some risk of infection. However, much may be done to minimise the risk. In hospitals in which patients are isolated in individual cubicles or wards, the danger of infection is minimised. The more patients are crowded together in an undivided ward, the greater the likelihood of case-to-case infection via the air.

Many hospitals which are still in use today were designed and built before the principles of infection were understood; infection is more likely in such old-fashioned buildings than in modern hospitals designed with a view to eliminating infection.

However, it is really the human beings who work in the hospital rather than the structure that make the decisive difference. A good staff in an old-fashioned hospital may keep the hospital free from avoidable infection, whereas the most modern buildings are no protection if the staff are slapdash in their methods and behaviour.

Air Infection

Air may be infected directly from the patients themselves, from their bedding or clothes, from bed curtains or from surgical dressings or instruments, or from the clothing or hands of nurses, doctors and other people in the ward.

Infection from Direct Contact

It is not only the air which may spread infection. It can spread from direct contact between patients, from contact with infected food, from cutlery and crockery, from linen, furniture and surgical instruments. It may spread from packs of surgical dressings if these are used after they have been contaminated. It may spread from bottles of lotion and ointments, even from bottles of disinfectants, if these are used first on an infected patient and then on others. The possibilities are endless.

However, there is no need for any feeling that the task of suppressing infection is hopeless or even particularly formidable. It is not. All that is needed is a sound understanding of a few basic principles, and common sense. More than anything else, common sense is important in the control of infection within hospitals.

Not only patients may become infected, but also nurses and doctors, physiotherapists, radiologists, domestics, porters and orderlies. If their infection is undetected they may spread it to others including patients. If it is detected they may have to undergo treatment, and go off work. Either event can lead to serious difficulties. So it is one of the duties of a nurse, or anyone else looking after patients, to avoid infection themselves as much as they can. This is an important part of their job.

During the course of training nurses and others should acquire habits of work which avoid infection, so that the correct behaviour becomes second nature to them, and they know instinctively what to do and what to avoid doing.

Some Patients are Especially Vulnerable

While it is possible for any patients to contract infection in hospitals, not all patients are equally vulnerable. It is obvious that some have more resistance than others, and some are particularly liable to pick up any infection that is around on account of their weak condition.

Patients who are particularly liable to infection are:
1. Newborn infants.
2. Premature babies.
3. Mothers during labour.
4. Surgical patients, especially while operations or dressings are in

progress, or whose wounds are exposed for other reasons, or patients with extensive burns.

5. Patients with deep-seated systemic diseases such as endocrine disorders, malignant disease, and leukaemia.
6. Patients on steroids, immunosuppressive, and anti-metabolite drugs.
7. Patients undergoing renal dialysis.
8. Patients immobilised for orthopaedic reasons.

In the Wards

Everything possible should be done to prevent the transference of microbes from patient to patient. The best way to do this is to keep the wards clean. Floors and walls should be washed regularly. The intervals between washes vary from hospital to hospital and depend on the staff available. Moreover, some kinds of surface get dirty more quickly than others. Hospitals in cities usually need more frequent washing than hospitals in country districts. While soap and water are often adequate for this purpose a disinfectant is more effective (see Chapter 9). Lockers, tables, trolleys and chairs should also be washed regularly.

Open wounds on surgical patients should only be exposed when the air of the ward is relatively undisturbed. The worst time to do dressings is when

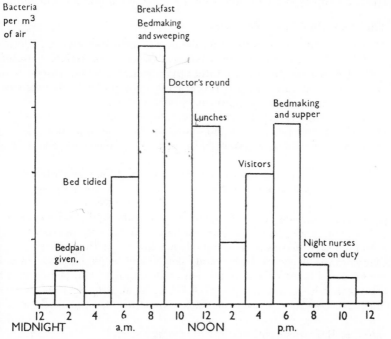

Fig. 28. The effect of activity on the bacterial content of air in a hospital ward

beds are being made, or just afterwards. A busy ward round, especially if the doctors are accompanied by students, is also the cause of much air disturbance which may lead to infection of any exposed wounds. The effect of various kinds of activity on the bacterial content of the air of wards is shown in Figure 28. Obviously, dressings should be done at times when air contamination is at its lowest.

Sweeping, cleaning and dusting should all have been completed before dressings are started. Better still, all ward cleaning should be done by vacuum cleaners with impermeable bags, to prevent the scattering of dust.

The design of the wards makes a lot of difference to the practicability of keeping down hospital infection. Large open wards are obviously more likely to favour cross-infection than the smaller wards which are found in most modern hospitals. This is a matter beyond the control of the nurse, who has to do the best work possible under the conditions in which she finds herself. However, the movement of beds in open wards, and the spaces between them, are often left to the discretion of the sister in charge, and can have a great effect on the transference of infection.

The correct space between bed centres is eight feet or more. This space cannot be achieved in many old-fashioned hospitals, but it is one that should be aimed at. The corridor between the rows of beds should be as wide as possible; ten to twelve feet is the minimum. The temptation to place an extra bed in the middle of the ward should be resisted; this often acts as a stepping stone for infection from one side of the ward to another.

The Operating Theatre—Asepsis

All surgery today is performed on the *aseptic* principle, that is, microbes should be excluded from the site of surgical procedures. Asepsis is a subject that is best learned in practice rather than from textbooks; a week or two of work in an operating theatre is worth any amount of book knowledge. It is also to a large extent a matter of common sense.

The entire operating theatre suite should be regarded as a special place to be kept as free from microbes as possible. Dust and dirt should be kept to a minimum, and unnecessary traffic of people, trolleys and goods should be avoided.

Of course, the actual rules to be adopted may differ slightly in different theatres. Some theatre suites are old-fashioned or badly designed, so that rules which may well be effective in modern suites would be ineffective in them. None the less, the same general principles hold good everywhere and the elimination of unnecessary dust and dirt will help in every theatre

In modern theatre suites, everybody has to wear clothing different from that worn in the rest of the hospital. This should be put on when entering the suite and taken off before it is left. All clothing should be put on, and taken off, with the minimum of shaking, as shaking scatters bacteria Ordinary shoes should never come into contact with the theatre floor; they often carry spore-bearing organisms. Overboots must be worn over outdoor shoes, or shoes taken off and theatre boots put on.

In the theatres themselves, it is even more important to keep out dust hence keeping down airborne infection. Even when operations are not in progress people should not enter the theatres without good cause, and the doors should be kept closed. Between operating lists, as much clean air as possible should be admitted, in order to flush out the theatres. If the air intake is filtered, it is a good plan to run the ventilation system at top speed for some hours before starting the day's work.

Patients should not be brought into the theatre on the ward trolleys or in their ward clothes and bedding; these bring in infected dust. They should be transferred to another trolley in a special area outside the theatre.

Trays of instruments and liquids such as sterile water should not be left exposed for long periods before an operation list, as they may get infected by the movements of bringing a patient into the theatre.

During operation lists, no discipline can be too rigorous. No one should enter the theatre without over-boots or theatre boots, a sterile gown, a mask and a cap. Movements should be unhurried and deliberate; sudden rushes are more likely to scatter microbes, as well as distracting the surgeons. Any talking should be restricted to the giving of necessary instructions or information. Coughing should be avoided. Hands, arms and gowns should not be waved. There should be the minimum of moving about the theatre to get instruments and dressings. This means that the likely needs of the surgeon must be foreseen, and the instruments and apparatus which might possibly be required should be got ready in a convenient place as near to the operating table as possible. A calm and unhurried atmosphere makes not only for the avoidance of infection but for good surgery; its maintenance is almost entirely a matter of the personalities of the theatre sister and of the surgeon. Mopping the surgeon's brow can be a dangerous action (though not to do so may be even more dangerous!). If this is necessary, the surgeon should turn right away from the operation site and his brow should be mopped with as little movement as possible.

No one should enter, or leave, a theatre during an operation list without good reason. Messengers should be firmly discouraged, or forbidden entirely. Any messages to people in theatre can be relayed by a radio, telephone or speaker system which should be discreet enough not to disturb the surgeons. In an experiment in one operating theatre it was shown that the number of infected cases was reduced by about 90 per cent simply by preventing people from entering, or leaving, the theatre unnecessarily.

During the progress of an operation, one must distinguish between the 'sterile' and 'non-sterile' sides of the theatre. The former includes the operation site, the top operation towels, the top covers of the operation trolleys and instrument tables. All else is non-sterile, and nothing which has been in contact with the latter should be allowed to the sterile side without being re-sterilised.

Scrubbing Up

If a nurse has to assist at an operation, either with the preparation of instruments, or at the actual operation site, she has to 'scrub-up'. The recommended technique differs according to whether disinfectants are used or not. The basic aim is always the same — to remove as many as possible of the bacteria from the surface of the hands. Sometimes a surface film of disinfectant is applied to the hands in a special soap.

Washing or scrubbing the hands for an operation should be done in a systematic manner. First the nails should be washed, then the backs of the hands and fingers, then the webs between the fingers at the back, finally the front of the hands and fingers. Then the hands should be rinsed. The nails should be kept short, and no nail varnish used.

A similar technique is used in the wards when scrubbing up for dressings.

Masks are used for two purposes. Their usual function is to prevent bacteria from reaching susceptible people from the respiratory tract of the wearer. An effective mask deflects the expired air sideways. Unfortunately many masks, for example, those made purely of cotton, are not very effective; some are only about 10 per cent effective. It is doubtful whether there is any point in using masks made entirely of cotton, no matter how many layers thick. Surgeons, and others, sometimes complain that effective masks feel oppressive. This is, without doubt, often the case, but there is no sense in wearing an ineffective mask simply because it feels comfortable.

Recent work has thrown doubt upon the value of using masks in hospital wards for surgical dressings. They should, however, be used in operating theatres, labour wards and premature baby units.

The second purpose of a mask is to protect the wearer, for instance, when nursing patients with open tuberculosis.

Infants' Nurseries

Newborn infants are extremely susceptible to infection. The eyes, the umbilicus and the skin ('septic spots') are especially vulnerable; any of these may be the seat of staphylococcal or other infection. Such infection is usually trivial, though it may lead to serious illness and septicaemia. Staphylococcal pneumonia is always serious and may be fatal.

On the other hand, a baby may spread microbes to nurses and doctors, and hence to other babies. So far as infection is concerned, every infant should be regarded in two ways — both as particularly vulnerable, and as a potentially dangerous spreader of microbes to others.

The danger of spreading infection from babies can be minimised in various ways. A long moist umbilical cord, for example, can be the source of much trouble. If cords are kept short and dry there is little danger of spread of infection from this source. Also, babies who show the slightest signs of infection — runny eyes, septic spots — should be taken out of the communal nursery whenever possible and put into rooms by themselves.

Dressing Techniques

Surgical dressings are 'taken down' and changed for two reasons. The first is to enable the surgeons and nurses to inspect the wound to see how it is getting on. The second is to clean the wound and so facilitate healing. Discharge, debris, pus and necrotic material hinder healing, and should be removed. The actively growing cells of a healing surface are extremely sensitive and tender; the wound should be dressed with the utmost gentleness. Fresh dressing materials with, or without, suitable medicaments should be applied, and the wound covered again to protect it from the outside world.

Exposing a wound, however, is dangerous; it makes infection possible as the raw surface unprotected by skin is a good culture medium for microbes. If a wound is exposed for inspection or dressing the net result may be harmful to the patient. For this reason dressings are done as infrequently as possible today, and more reliance than in the past is placed on the natural processes of healing. A clean wound is best left undisturbed.

Sometimes, where there is much discharge, or a drainage tube has been used, frequent dressings are unavoidable.

All dressing materials should be set out in such a way as to reduce the likelihood of contaminating them. The dressings and instruments used, should, of course, all be sterile. They may be sterilised on the wards or, as is common today, in a central sterilising department (see below). They should be laid out on the trolley in a manner which will not contaminate them. Two nurses are needed to do a dressing properly—one 'sterile' nurse and one 'dirty' nurse. Before doing the dressing the 'sterile' nurse should scrub up. Strict 'no-touch' technique should be used. Care should be taken that sterile dressings and instruments are not contaminated by contact with soiled ones or with unsterile hands. All soiled dressings should be placed in a disposable bag, and soiled instruments in another bag.

The bags should be kept closed to prevent their contents from spreading infection.

These aseptic precautions should always be taken when a wound is to be exposed. Surgeons and nurses should never handle wounds without carefully washing their hands first.

Dressings should never be done in the ward while the ward is being cleaned, or while beds are being made. Time should be allowed for the dust to settle after such activities.

Dressing Rooms

The best way to avoid wound contamination during dressings is to do the dressings, not in the ward, but in a special 'dressing room' reserved for this purpose. Such rooms are to be found in modern hospitals, but in most older hospitals dressings still have to be done in the wards.

The actual technique of dressings is set out in books and articles devoted to the subject. It is a technique which can only be learned by experience.

Central Sterile Supply Departments (CSSD)

A comparatively recent change in many hospitals has been the introduction of Central Sterile Supply Departments (CSSD). Formerly, dressings or packs were made up by nurses in the wards. Nowadays, packs of sterile supplies for use in the wards are made up and sterilised in a special department of the hospital designed and staffed for this purpose — a small factory within the hospital. The CSSD thus liberates the nursing staff from much tedious work in the manufacture of dressings, and enables them to spend their working hours doing their proper job, which is the care of patients.

Some CSSD also supply the hospital operating theatres, though these sometimes prefer to make up their own packs.

Most CSSDs supply a variety of packs. These are broadly of four types:

1. Packs containing a number of articles used in almost every procedure, such as cotton wool balls, gauze swabs.

2. More elaborate packs 'tailor-made' for particular procedures such as lumbar punctures.

3. Packs of sterile instruments.

4. Specialised packs for uncommon procedures, or made to suit the requirements of particular surgeons, are also prepared.

The packs are made up by specially trained staff, and sterilised in autoclaves in the CSSD. Thence they are distributed to the wards.

There are several different methods of distributing sterile supplies; each hospital has its particular method suited to its particular problems of work-load and hospital geography. In some hospitals, the ward sister sends a written requisition for sterile goods, on a special form, to the CSSD the day before they are required. In others the 'topping up' or 'grocery van' system, a trolley from the CSSD makes a daily round to the wards topping up the ward list of requirements.

For a CSSD to operate successfully, the following are essential:

1. Intelligent anticipation by the nursing staff of their likely requirements.

2. Since this anticipation cannot be exact, and emergencies constantly arise, there must be proper provision by the CSSD for speedy emergency supplies to the wards. Sometimes this takes the form of an emergency store or cupboard situated near the CSSD, the key to which is obtainable by ward sisters during hours when the CSSD is closed.

3. Collaboration and co-operation between the nursing staff and the CSSD staff. This is essential. A good CSSD with a keen superintendent is a priceless asset to any hospital. But for close working between the CSSD and the ward there must be mutual confidence between them. The ward staff must feel that they can rely on regular and reliable supplies, otherwise they will naturally tend to 'hoard' supplies. The CSSD must feel that they are trusted to deliver the goods and that goods are not being unnecessarily wasted. A certain amount of wastage is of course inevitable if patients are to be properly looked after. It is not necessary or possible that every last gauze swab or cotton wool ball should be accounted for. But sterile packs, which cost money to make up, sterilise, and deliver, should not be wasted unnecessarily any more than anything else.

To get the most benefit out of sterile supplies, new dressing techniques may have to be devised to take account of the way in which packs are made up. It is obviously essential to prepare packs so that they may be quickly laid out in an aseptic manner. This requires a lot of close co-operation between ward sister and CSSD superintendent, first in working out the contents of each pack, secondly in working out a way of folding and packing the pack, and thirdly in working out a way in unfolding it and setting it out in the wards.

A good CSSD supervisor must have a combination of unusual qualities. He or she must have some knowledge of surgery and of nursing, especially of dressing techniques. He or she must be an expert on sterilisation procedures and on the workings of modern autoclaves. He or she should have some idea of factory management and labour relations. He or she must be patient, courteous, and able to get on well with theatre sisters, surgeons, and hospital administrators.

It is always a good thing if, during their training period, student nurses spend some time in the CSSD to see how packs are made up and sterilised. Apart from anything else, this is likely to give them an idea of the amount of thinking and of work involved in preparing packs, and so reduce the likelihood of wastage when they use packs in the wards.

Packing Materials

Packs are made up of a convenient selection of articles, wrapped for sterilisation and storage in such a way that they may be unpacked and used while yet remaining sterile. In general, this means that they have to be double-wrapped. The outside wrapping is regarded as unsterile on the outside but sterile on the inside. The inner wrapping is completely sterile, as of course are the contents.

A wide variety of fabrics, such as linens and special types of paper, have been devised for wrapping packs. Polythene is unsuitable for packs which are sterilised in autoclaves, as it is not penetrated by steam. Polythene is, however, much used for packs which are sterilised by irradiation.

The wrapped packs are usually placed for sterilisation into cardboard boxes with deep sides. These may be sterilised safely a number of times. Each box should have a record on it on which is noted each time it is packed, sterilised, and opened. Such boxes have now superseded the old metal drums, which were unreliable, noisy, and heavy.

Sterile goods in boxes or packs often have to be stored in the wards. They should be stored either in closed cupboards or drawers, not on open shelves where they may be contaminated by dust thereby endangering the contents.

It is important that sterile supplies are used in rotation, the oldest being used first. In good storage conditions, supplies remain sterile for a long time but not for an indefinite time.

Isolation of Patients

In isolating patients our knowledge of the value of many of the measures in general use is very incomplete. No one yet knows for certain how effective are many of the precautions taken to prevent the spread of infection to or from patients. What has been attempted here is to give a common sense guide to reasonable practice.

Patients may be isolated for the following reasons:

1. To protect other people from their microbes (source isolation).
2. To protect them from infection (protective isolation).

These must be distinguished.

1. *Source Isolation*

In recent years there has been a big change in views about isolating infected patients, and there is still a lot of difference of opinion about its value. In theory, of course, every patient who is a source of microbes dangerous to others should be nursed at a safe distance from other patients, so as to reduce the possibility of microbes travelling from the infectious to the susceptible patient. In the past, there was little precise knowledge about the likelihood of particular microbes spreading from patient to patient. Until quite recently, hospitals were constructed on the principle that nearly all types of infection could travel long distances. Infectious diseases hospitals had wards in isolated buildings, in each of which a different disease was often housed. Such a method of construction has obvious disadvantages in that the hospital with wards widely spread out presents serious problems of transport and the provision of hot meals and so on.

Nowadays we have much more precise knowledge about how infections are spread. Some diseases, such as measles, are extremely infectious, and no one can reasonably doubt the value of isolating cases, and allowing only people who are immune to come into contact with the patient. Other diseases, such as streptococcal tonsillitis and scarlet fever, are much less infectious. Though isolation is desirable, it is possible to nurse these cases in a general ward provided the specific dangers are understood and the necessary precautionary measures taken. The development of antibiotics has made it much easier to nurse patients with streptococcal infections. Immunisation has so reduced the incidence of diphtheria that this has now become a rare disease. In many countries, such as Great Britain, only sporadic cases occur, instead of the large numbers regularly encountered thirty years ago. In such countries, diphtheria wards are now obsolete. Indeed, infectious diseases hospitals are much less used today, and many have been converted to other uses.

None the less, most infectious patients should still be isolated if possible, and in some infections this is essential. The tendency today, wherever possible, is to isolate patients in separate air-conditioned rooms in compact buildings instead of herding those with a particular disease into a large ward in an isolated building. What can actually be done in any particular hospital depends on its structure and the nature of the wards. There are still some hospitals with few isolation rooms or cubicles. In such hospitals, infectious cases cannot be nursed at all with reasonable safety, and the patients should be transferred to a hospital for infectious diseases.

The Nursing of Patients with Bowel Infections

Entirely different considerations arise when we are dealing with patients suffering from bowel infections, such as typhoid, paratyphoid, bacterial food poisoning, salmonella, or dysentery. Here the means of infection is by the faeces of a patient and by his urine. The mouth and nasal secretions and the sputum of such patients are not infectious. The danger lies in the utensils, cutlery, crockery, food leavings, urinals, bedpans, and bed-clothes. While undoubtedly full isolation in a separate room or cubicle is ideal, none the less in general these patients need a lesser degree of isolation than that required for those who spread airborne diseases. A corner of a general ward may be adequate.

The faeces and vomit of these patients contains dangerous microbes. Care should be taken in handling these, especially when the patient has liquid faeces which are liable to be splashed about. Patients should wash their hands in disinfectant solution after defaecating. Their cutlery and crockery should be kept separate from those of the other patients in the ward and disinfected after use. Their bedlinen should be regarded as fouled, and dealt with specially as described (page 100).

Nurses should wash their hands after handling these patients, their bedclothes, or their bedpans or vomit-bowls.

Some diseases are spread both by airborne spread by droplet infection and by faecal contamination. Poliomyelitis and infective hepatitis are both spread in this way. However, the likelihood of either of these diseases being conveyed to other people is a great deal less than that of many other infectious fevers listed above. The nursing of such patients in general wards depends on scrupulous technique and undoubtedly always places a great strain on the nurses. This is also true of the bowel infections already mentioned.

Ideally, every patient who is regarded as infectious should be removed to a separate room or cubicle, and 'cubicle' means a room with its own door, window and wash basin, and in which the walls go right up to the ceiling. It should have independent ventilation so that there is little danger of infected air reaching other patients.

In addition to the physical removal of infectious patients, other measures can be taken to reduce the risk of infection. The first is to wear **protective clothing**. A gown or plastic apron should be put on before the nurse or other attendant goes near the patient to carry out any nursing procedure, or disturb the bedclothes. It should be taken off when she leaves. Care should be taken, when putting on or taking off this garment, not to scatter microbes about. If possible, it should be put on and taken off in a special ante-room.

Gowns should be sent for sterilising and laundering after every day's use. Plastic aprons should be washed down daily with a disinfectant (see Chapter 9).

Infectivity

The most rational approach to the question of isolating patients is through a consideration of their infectivity, that is to say, the way in which infection is likely to spread from them to other patients.

For patients with diseases of the respiratory passages, this is likely to be by droplet infection carried through the air. These patients should *always* be isolated in separate rooms or cubicles. So should cases of fevers with infective skin rashes, the exanthemata. **Patients with the following diseases should be transferred to an infectious diseases unit as soon as possible:**

Bacillary dysentery	Paratyphoid
Chicken-pox	Poliomyelitis
Cholera	Rubella
Diphtheria	Salmonella infection
Herpes zoster	Smallpox
Infantile diarrhoea	'Open' tuberculosis
Measles	Typhoid
Mumps	Whooping cough

Droplets of secretion from these patients may attach themselves to the clothing of an attendant, so that nurses and doctors who look after these patients should put on a gown and take it off again before they enter another ward or the general hospital circulation space.

2. *Protective Isolation — Isolation of Vulnerable Patients*

Patients are isolated not only because they are a danger to others, but because they are particularly vulnerable to infections. Examples of such patients are listed on pages 88-9.

All these patients should be nursed in single rooms or cubicles wherever possible. Specially designed isolation units are sometimes built for this purpose. Babies may be nursed in a common nursery provided care is taken to avoid contact between cots.

Various elaborate ways of isolation are being tried out in hospitals throughout the world. Among them may be mentioned **Ultra-clean units**, in which patients are nursed in aseptic conditions resembling those in use in operating theatres. Another method of isolating is by use of a **Mobile Isolator**. This consists essentially of a large transparent plastic tent, as big as a cubicle, inside which a patient may be isolated while he can still see what is going on in the ward around him and is still in view of nurses and doctors outside the isolator.

Surveillance of Ward Staff

Whenever vulnerable patients are being nursed, it is necessary to have frequent checks of the infectivity of ward staffs. In practice, this usually means that they are checked to see whether or not they are carrying staphylococci. **Nasal swabs** and **hand swabs** are frequently taken, either once or twice a week. Nasal swabs should be taken from the anterior nares.

Nurses, doctors, and domestic staff should all be included in this routine swabbing.

When a member of staff is found to carry staphylococci, he or she should be treated. Perhaps the most effective way of doing this is by means of an antiseptic spray which the carrier is instructed to use several times a day.

In some wards, all staff regularly use antiseptic sprays whether or not their nasal swabs are positive.

Barrier Nursing

A time-honoured method of isolating patients in wards with or without isolation in separate rooms or cubicles is by barrier nursing. This usually consists of the following:

1. **Isolation** of the patient in a separate room or cubicle, or, when this is not possible, in a remote corner of the ward behind screens.

2. **Protective clothing**. Gowns or aprons are put on, near the bedside, by nurses or doctors attending the patient. They are taken off as soon as the doctor or nurse leaves the patient. Gowns are replaced every day and plastic aprons are washed with, or dipped in, disinfectants daily.

3. **Masks** may also be used by nurses or doctors.

4. **Hand washing**. Where a separate hand basin is not available close to the patient's bed, a bowl of disinfectant solution is kept by the bedside for the nurse or doctor to wash their hands in after looking after the patient.

5. **Cutlery and crockery**. Separate feeding utensils are kept for the patient, and are disinfected, separate from the other ward cutlery and crockery, after use.

6. **Bedlinen** is put into an infected laundry bag, and is separately disinfected after use.

7. **Mattresses and pillows**. If kept in plastic covers, these are swabbed with a disinfectant solution at regular intervals, and on discharge of the patient. Others are disinfected by autoclaving by formalin, or by baking in an oven.

The effectiveness of barrier nursing depends on how well it is done. When the general standards of nursing is very good, it plays an important part in preventing the spread of infection.

Barrier nursing in an open ward should still be practised where there are no facilities for full isolation. Undoubtedly, isolation in a separate room or cubicle is better where there are facilities for it.

Terminal Disinfection

This means the disinfection of the bedding and clothing of an infected patient after he or she has been discharged from the hospital or has died. **Mattresses** are difficult to disinfect, and the method used depends on the type of mattress. Some can be heated in ovens, others may have to be treated with formaldehyde vapour at low temperatures.

Linen

Handling soiled bedlinen is a possible way of spreading microbes. Sorting such linen for the laundry invariably scatters microbes into the atmosphere and increases the chances of infection.

All used linen should be removed from the ward as soon as possible. It should be put into impermeable bags, and taken away uncounted.

Any linen that is particularly badly soiled, for example with faeces, or linen from patients with such diseases as typhoid, other salmonella infections or dysentery, should be regarded as 'fouled' and soaked in a liquid disinfectant. This should preferably be done outside the ward, after the linen has been removed in specially marked closed impermeable bags.

Laundries

In most laundries, cotton goods are boiled; this kills vegetative bacteria but not spore bearers. Woollen goods such as blankets cannot be boiled without reducing their effective life. A cold antiseptic wash should be used for these. Nowadays the tendency in hospitals is to substitute cotton blankets, or those made with man-made fibres, for woollen ones.

Laundry bags should be made of some material which can be sterilised. Cotton or nylon are suitable; they can be closed with zip fasteners, or tied with tapes. Wicker baskets should never be used as they cannot be effectively sterilised.

Where the hospital has its own laundry, the laundering process can be effectively supervised. Supervision is much more difficult where a commercial laundry is used. None the less it is important that the hospital authorities retain some control over the processes used. It is also important in safeguarding the general public who are the other customers of the laundry. They do not want to have their linen soiled by contact with that from the hospital.

The Prevention of Food-borne Infection

It is important for nurses to have a good knowledge of the principles of food hygiene; they are often responsible for supervising catering staff, or for looking after or serving food in hospital wards, institutions, or private homes.

Food-borne infection is due to the contamination of food or drink. The main sources of this are:

1. The **faeces** of an infected person, either directly, or indirectly, via the **hands**, or objects which have been handled. This can be prevented by personal hygiene. Everyone should wash his hands after passing urine or faeces. Unfortunately, this is not quite as simple as it sounds, for there may be no facilities for doing so. These should be available everywhere, and in public lavatories they should be free of charge. The very young and infirm

may not be able to wash after defaecating. They should have it done for them.

2. **Sewage**, through the use of infected water supplies.

3. **Flies**, which may infect food after contact with sewage, refuse dumps, dustbins, or exposed faeces. Flies should be kept down by abolishing exposed collections of refuse and by the use of insecticides.

4. The **hands** of people who handle food, whether in the home, in restaurants, shops, or food-factories. Food should be handled as little as possible. It should not be handled by those who have to handle money in shops, who should use tongs, or alternatively all the food should be wrapped before handling.

5. The **air**, through infected dust.

6. **Domestic animals and pets**, which may spread salmonella infection.

In a kitchen or food shop or restaurant, one infected article of food may contaminate others, either directly or via utensils and slicing machines, etc.

The most important microbes concerned in food poisoning are:

1. **Staphylococci** – from the hands, hair or airborne infection. These may multiply in the food, producing enterotoxin, so that food poisoning occurs when the food is eaten.

2. **Salmonellas** – especially *S. typhi-murium* and *S. enteritidis*. These come from faeces, contaminated hands, flies, or domestic animals and pets.

3. **Coliform bacilli** – from the same sources as salmonellas.

4. **Pseudomonas** – from the same sources, from the air.

5. **Clostridium welchii** – from dust or dirt, which may also multiply in food and produce a toxin.

So far as food preparation is concerned, the golden rule is — **Keep it cool; keep it clean; keep it covered.**

It goes without saying that all the raw materials of food, including the water supply, must be clean and uninfected.

Food must be cooked as soon as possible after preparation. If it has to wait before cooking, it must be kept in a refrigerator. Food should never be allowed to stand at room temperature. It must be served under clean conditions. Unused remains should be covered promptly and put into a refrigerator if they are to be used again. Food which is reheated after standing at room temperature is an important source of food poisoning.

All who are concerned in the serving and preparation of food — domestic staff, cooks, and servers — must observe rigorous personal hygiene. Hands must be washed before starting work and after going to the lavatory. Finger nails must be kept clean and short. Hair must be clean and is best covered by a cap, hat or scarf. Overalls and aprons must be clean.

No one with clinical sepsis of any kind should be allowed to handle or serve food. Even a small staphylococcal lesion on the hands may spread millions of dangerous organisms. No one with any sort of bowel upset should be allowed into a kitchen, nor should they serve meals.

The kitchen and all the equipment — utensils, crockery, tables, ventilators, and so on—must be clean. Kitchen floors and walls must be washed frequently. Dustbins must be kept covered.

Cutlery and Crockery

Whenever possible, infectious patients should have their own cutlery and crockery which is disinfected by heat or disinfectants after use. If all the ward crockery and cutlery is treated in this way in any case, for example, in a washing-up machine operated at over 80 ° C, then no other special precautions are necessary.

Toothmugs

Mugs used by patients for cleaning their teeth or leaving their dentures in overnight are a possible source of cross-infection. Mugs should be washed daily, and every patient should have his own. Better still, disposable ones should be issued and used once only.

Clinical Thermometers

There should be a separate thermometer for each patient, which should be kept in disinfectant solution (see Chapter 9) when it is not in use. When the patient has been discharged, the thermometer should be thoroughly washed before being issued to another patient.

Urinals

Urinals should be disinfected after use. They should then be stored in a stand in which they are not liable to pick up infection. They should be issued to patients in fresh paper bags. On no account should they be issued covered with a cloth that is used many times; this is a dangerous source of infection. After use they can be returned to the sluice room in the same paper bags which are then thrown away.

Disposable urinals are available, and do away with the need for disinfection. However, they are expensive and take up a lot of valuable storage space.

Bedpans

Bedpans, after use, should be emptied and steamed or thoroughly washed with hot water, preferably in a machine designed for the purpose. They should then be stored in a cabinet in which they will not pick up infection. They should be issued to the patient in fresh paper bags in which they can be returned after use. The bags should then be thrown away.

Disposable bedpans are available, which are destroyed after use in a pulverising machine plumbed to the drainage system. They have to be placed on a plastic stand for use by the patient; the stand does not normally get soiled, though it should be washed with disinfectant every time it is used.

Disposable bedpans take up a lot of storage space.

It is important that bedpan washing and disposal machines are kept in good working order by effective maintenance. Otherwise they may help to spread infection.

CHAPTER 9

STERILISATION AND DISINFECTION

Many terms are rather loosely used in discussing sterilisation. What follows are a few working definitions (see also Glossary, page 163).

Sterilisation means the destruction of all living microbes, and incidentally of all other living matter.

Disinfection means the destruction of all vegetative microbes, that is to say, excluding spores.

A **bacteriostatic agent** is one which prevents microbes from multiplying, but does not necessarily kill them.

Germicide means the same as disinfectant.

An **antiseptic** is a substance which is applied locally to prevent infection, either by killing microbes, or by preventing them from multiplying.

Methods of sterilisation fall into two groups: (a) **Physical** and (b) **Chemical**.

(a) Physical Methods of Disinfection

    1. Sunlight and ultra-violet light.
    2. Heat.
       (i) Hot water sterilisers
      (ii) Hot air ovens
    (iii) Infra red heating
    (iv) Microwave ovens
     (v) Steam methods — autoclaves and pressure cookers
    3. Irradiation.

1. Sunlight

Direct exposure to the rays of the sun will eventually kill all living things. Sunlight as a disinfectant can have appreciable effects. For example, the play of sunlight on the surface of an open-air swimming pool does kill some bacteria and signifies that, other things being equal, open-air pools are likely to contain less microbes than enclosed pools. Hanging the washing out in the sun sterilises it as well as drying it. The obvious advantage of sterilising by sunlight, where and when available, is that it costs nothing.

It is the ultra-violet rays of the sun which exert the lethal effect, and the same effect can be achieved artificially by use of an ultra-violet lamp. Such a lamp is often used to sterilise bottles of biological fluids, such as blood or plasma, which cannot be conveniently sterilised in any other way. Ultra-violet rays can also be used in the form of a screen, to sterilise air entering a room. Many laboratories in which work requiring a high degree of sterility is performed have such ultra-violet screens. They are also used occasionally in operating theatres. Experiments have been done in schoolrooms to see whether the air can be kept relatively microbe-free by this means. In these experiments ultra-violet lamps were hung from the ceiling to sterilise the upper layers of the air. It was found that school-children using these classrooms had a lower rate of respiratory disease than children using untreated classrooms in the same school, presumably because the numbers of microbes were reduced in the air of the treated rooms.

It must, of course, be remembered that excessive exposure to ultra-violet light is very dangerous to human beings. When objects are being sterilised by ultra-violet light, exposure of the human body, especially the eyes, to the rays must be avoided, by protective clothing, by wearing goggles, and so on.

Another disadvantage of ultra-violet irradiation or sunlight as a disinfectant is that to be effective it must act directly on the object to be sterilised. Dirt may prevent ultra-violet rays from reaching the object to be sterilised. The rays will not penetrate ordinary glass.

2. Heat

The physical means of sterilisation which is used more than any other is the application of heat. This can be applied in any number of ways, of which the following are the most important:

(i) Hot Water Sterilisers

The easiest way of applying heat is by heating water in a kettle or a hot-water steriliser. Such sterilisers used to be a feature of all hospital wards and operating theatres, but they are now disappearing as quickly as central sterilising departments are installed in hospitals. The highest temperature obtainable in an open vessel is 100 °C. At this temperature, the water evaporates and turns to steam. Until all the water has evaporated, the temperature will remain steady at 100 °C. On escaping from the vessel, the steam immediately condenses back into water, producing clouds of droplets which heat and dampen the atmosphere, often making it very difficult to work, and incidentally, spreading infection.

Effectiveness

How effective is hot water as a sterilising agent? **All viruses and all vegetative, that is, non-sporing, bacteria are killed in a few seconds by temperatures well below that of boiling water.** 60 °C is hot enough to kill most of them, though some can survive 80° C. Spores, however, are another matter. All spores need higher temperatures to kill them than do vegetative bacteria. Some can resist boiling for several hours, though this is exceptional. None the less, to be quite sure that microbes of all kinds have been killed, boiling should continue for six hours.

This is, of course, quite impracticable, and indeed it is unnecessary when one is only trying to kill vegetative microbes, as may be the case when one is 'scalding out' a baby's feeding bottle in the home. This 'scalding out' is not really sterilisation. In the circumstances of the home it may be adequate, however, as the danger to the baby comes mostly from the vegetative organisms, which cause bowel infections, rather than from spore-bearers.

However, all surgical instruments and clothing must be sterilised. If it is necessary to sterilise instruments during an operating list, some other method than boiling should be used; for example, a rapidly acting auto-clave. The practice of boiling instruments for a few minutes between operations is inadequate and unsafe. It will dispose of vegetative organisms but not of the spore-bearers, which are potentially dangerous in surgery.

(ii) Hot-Air Ovens

The conventional gas or electric hot-air oven can be used over a wide range of temperatures. The higher the temperature, the less the exposure time needed to kill spores. The usual temperature is 160 °C, in which all sporing organisms are killed in forty-five minutes. Hot air is not as effective as steam, and a temperature hot enough to kill spores will damage most fabrics and will eventually damage rubber and plastics. Linen, cotton, cotton-wool, and other fabrics cannot, therefore, be sterilised in this way. This severely limits the use of the method, which, however, is useful for syringes in metal and glass containers, and glass or metal apparatus.

Another disadvantage is the long time taken for most ovens to heat up and cool down again, often as long as or longer than the actual sterilising time of forty-five minutes. So the objects to be sterilised have to be in the oven for about two hours in all. Most homes have an oven in the kitchen, however, which means that this kind of sterilising can be performed almost anywhere by general practitioners and private nurses.

(iii) Infra-Red Heating

The infra-red end of the spectrum consists of rays which give no visible light but much heat. These can be directed on to objects to sterilise them from a suitable source such as a lamp. A high temperature of 180 °C or more can be attained which has to be held only for about ten minutes; this short sterilising time is a big advantage of infra-red heating. Another advantage is that the heating does not have to be done in a confined and insulated space such as an oven. A moving conveyor belt passing under an infra-red lamp is a convenient way of using this form of sterilisation, and is often used for sterilising syringes in a syringe unit.

(iv) Micro-Wave Ovens

In this, heating to the desired temperature takes a matter of seconds only. However, the temperature of micro-wave ovens is uneven, and while some parts of the object may be effectively sterilised, other parts may not be. The addition of infra-red heating to a micro-wave oven gets over this difficulty.

(v) **Autoclave**

The most important method of sterilising used in hospitals is by means of steam under pressure, in an **Autoclave**.

How an autoclave works

Steam is a more effective steriliser than hot air, and steam at 120 °C will kill all living objects in fifteen minutes. This temperature is attained by keeping the steam at a pressure greater than atmospheric pressure. If steam is fed into an autoclave from a boiler, and the interior of the autoclave sealed off from the outside, the temperature of the steam inside the autoclave can be maintained at the desired level indefinitely.

Autoclaves are complicated pieces of apparatus (see Fig. 29) and if they are to be used correctly it is necessary to understand how they work. The commonest mistake is to think that the temperature inside the autoclave is sufficient to sterilise on its own. This is not so. Only *steam* at this temperature is an effective sterilising agent in the time allowed; hot air at this temperature is not; it is not hot enough. It follows that for effective autoclave sterilising, the steam must actually reach the object to be sterilised and remain in contact with it for the required time. Moreover, the steam must be pure, not mixed with air. Any mixture with air reduces the effectiveness of the steam as a sterilising agent.

The first step in the use of the autoclave must, therefore, be the complete removal of the air. In modern 'high-vacuum' autoclaves, this is largely achieved by a powerful exhaust pump. In older 'downward displacement' autoclaves, the entering steam itself drives out the air. Air is heavier than steam, so if the steam is fed in from the top and there is an exhaust pipe for air at the bottom, the steam can drive out the air simply by coming in at the top. The air is forced out of the bottom by gravity.

At the end of the sterilising process, the air must be admitted once again to drive out the steam, before the temperature falls. Otherwise the steam will condense on the sterilised objects, and they will come out of the autoclave wet. This air must be filtered, or it may bring pathogenic microbes into the autoclave and contaminate the objects which have just been sterilised.

High-vacuum autoclaves take much less time to sterilise than do downward-displacement types, and on the whole they are more reliable. These are the main reasons why high-vacuum machines are replacing the latter. In the older type of autoclave it may take half-an-hour or more for the steam to enter the sterilising chamber and drive out all the air, before the actual sterilising begins. The sterilising time at a temperature of 120 °C

ITEM No.	DESCRIPTION
1	CHAMBER
2	STEAM JACKET
3	JACKET PRESSURE GAUGE
4	CHAMBER VAC. GAUGE
5	CHAMBER PRESSURE GAUGE
6	SAFETY VALVE
7	STEAM TO CHAMBER VALVE
8	AIR VALVE
9	AIR FILTER
10	REDUCING VALVE
11	GAUGE COCK & SYPHON
12	LINE PRESSURE GAUGE
13	STRAINER
14	MAIN STEAM VALVE
15	CONDENSATE CONNECTION
16	NON–RETURN VALVE
17	LINE STEAM TRAP
18	JACKET STEAM TRAP
19	THERMOCOUPLE CONNECTION
20	PROCESS MONITOR
21	TEST CONNECTION
22	EXHAUST VALVE
23	CONDENSATE REG. VALVE
24	CONDENSER
25	AIR EJECTOR
26	VACUUM PUMP
27	FEED TANK
28	BALL FLOAT VALVE
29	C.W. AUTO VALVE
30	DRAIN
31	DRAIN CONNECTION
32	C.W. STOP VALVE
33	DOOR CYLINDER

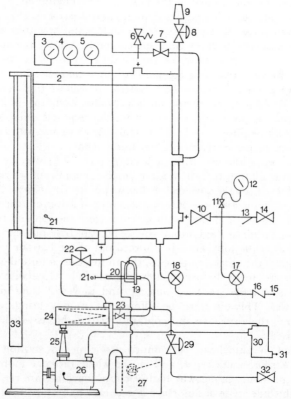

Fig. 29. Simplified (!) diagram of an autoclave. At least it shows how complicated this apparatus is

is twenty minutes. After sterilising, the steam must be driven out by air, and the temperature allowed to come down. This may take another half-hour, or more. A normal sterilising cycle may thus take almost two hours. This means that in a working day of eight hours, only four cycles can be got through.

In a high-vacuum autoclave the air is pumped out of the machine very quickly. The sterilising time is short as a higher temperature, usually about 136° C, is used than in a displacement machine. The steam is pumped out mechanically at the end. This means that the sterilising chamber can be made much smaller, and that it is economical to sterilise much smaller loads than in a displacement machine, in which the cycle takes just as long whether the sterilising chamber is full or nearly empty.

The whole cycle in a high-vacuum autoclave varies from a few minutes in small machines, to about thirty minutes in the largest types. So many more cycles can be got through in the course of a day.

A **pressure cooker** is a small steam steriliser. In it, however, there is no way of driving off the steam at the end of the sterilising process. Steam therefore condenses on the sterilised object as the cooker cools down, so that the contents emerge damp. When this does not matter, a pressure cooker is a convenient way of sterilising small objects.

What can be sterilised in an autoclave? Anything which can be reached by the steam under pressure, and which is not harmed by steam. All dressings, linen and cotton objects, and many types of instruments. However, they must be wrapped loosely, in such a way that the steam can penetrate them. The contents of impermeable packs such as polythene, or of glass containers with the caps screwed down, are *not* sterilised in an ordinary autoclave cycle. Other methods have to be used for these.

Assembled syringes cannot be sterilised in autoclaves either, as the steam will not penetrate into the interior. Syringes can only be sterilised in autoclaves when the plunger has been removed from the barrel. In this case, there is a danger of infecting the syringe when it is assembled for use. It is unsafe to use a syringe which has been assembled after being sterilised. So other methods than autoclaves have to be used for sterilising syringes, such as hot air in an oven, or irradiation.

It is surprising how often one sees polythene packs, assembled syringes, and screw-capped bottles placed in autoclaves for sterilising, by people who do not realise that the process is ineffective.

Testing autoclaves

The efficiency of autoclaves should be regularly tested—preferably every day. This can easily be done by various methods, of which the following are the best:

1. Thermophilic spores

Packets containing bacterial spores which are very heat resistant can be placed among the objects in the autoclave. After the sterilising cycle, they should be sent to the laboratory for culture. If they have been killed, it can be assumed that all other spores will have been killed also.

2. Browne's tubes

These are small sealed tubes containing chemicals which change colour

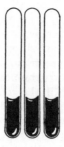

Fig. 30. Browne's tubes

at a definite temperature. Different tubes can be used for testing different types of steriliser. When the correct temperature is reached, they change from red to green; if it is not reached they remain a reddish-brown colour.

3. Heat-sensitive tape

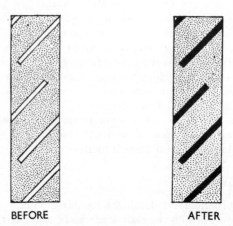

BEFORE   AFTER

Fig. 31. Heat-sensitive tape before and after sterilisation

Various types of tape are available in which a coloured pattern appears when the steam reaches the correct temperature. These can be used in the centre of a pile of goods (see below).

4. The Bowie-Dick test

In this test, which is probably the best test for autoclave efficiency, a diagonal cross of heat-sensitive tape is placed on a sheet of paper in the centre

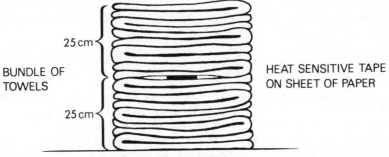

Fig. 32.   The Bowie-Dick test

towel of a standard sized pile of towels (50-55cm high). These are then put through a sterilising cycle in the autoclave. For the cycle to have been efficient, an even change of colour should have occurred in all parts of the tape.

TABLE OF STERILISING TIMES

Method	Temperatures (°C)	Sterilising time	Total sterilising cycle time
Hot water	100°	6 hours	6 hours (see p. 105)
Hot air: Conventional oven	160°	45 minutes	About 1½ hours
Infra-red oven	180°	5 minutes	10 minutes
Micro-wave		2 minutes	
Steam — Displacement autoclave	120°	20 minutes	About 2 hours (depending on size of autoclave)
High-vacuum autoclave	136°	5 minutes	About 20 minutes (depending on size of autoclave)

Irradiation (Ionizing Radiation)

Living objects may be killed by irradiation, or ionizing radiation, and this method is becoming increasingly used as a means of sterilisation. It would be possible to use the hospital radiotherapy apparatus for this purpose, but this is rarely practicable as the apparatus would need considerable adaptation. Specially designed apparatus is expensive, too expensive as a rule for an individual hospital. Moreover, those who use the method have to be carefully protected to prevent them from accidentally receiving a dose of radiation, which could be lethal. In practice, ionizing radiation is performed either by large commercial concerns or in government laboratories, using either:

1. Gamma radiation from cobalt-60, a highly radio-active substance, or
2. A linear accelerator (electron accelerator).

One advantage of irradiation sterilisation over heat methods is that there is no damage from heat. Another advantage is the superior penetration. High-energy electrons from a linear accelerator can penetrate a few centimetres, so this method of sterilisation is suitable only for small objects.

Gamma rays, on the other hand, can penetrate much further, through various types of packaging. Quite large sealed objects can be sterilised in this way, such as boxes of plastic syringes in polythene envelopes.

Some Ineffective Methods of Physical 'Sterilisation' — these are mentioned to prevent confusion.

(a) Cooling and refrigeration

Many people think that microbes can be killed by refrigerating them. While this is true of some bacteria it is not true of the majority and it is emphatically not true of viruses. In fact, the best way to preserve viruses alive is by refrigeration at very low temperatures such as $-20°C$; even lower temperatures are used. Food and other materials put in the refrigerator are not sterilised, no matter for how long the cooling takes place. On the other hand, the multiplication of bacteria is much reduced and may stop completely at refrigerator temperature.

(b) Drying

Again, drying is not a method of sterilisation. Some bacteria are killed by drying, but most are not.

Here it is perhaps worth mentioning that the best way of preserving bacteria and viruses alive is by a combination of the above methods — freeze-drying. Stock cultures of bacteria and smallpox and BCG vaccine are now commonly stored alive in sealed tubes after freeze-drying.

(c) Ultra-sonic vibrations

Ultra-sonic vibrations will eventually kill bacterial cells. However, the treatment has to be much more drastic than that usually carried out in ultra-sonic tanks used for cleaning apparatus. In these cleaning processes, some bacteria are killed but not all. So ultra-sonic methods as usually available in hospitals must be regarded as ineffective methods of sterilisation.

Chemical Disinfection

Chemicals have been used for disinfection for thousands of years, since long before people knew about the existence of microbes. In the Bible there are references to the use of wine and vinegar to preserve food and to prevent putrefaction. In every part of the world, chemicals of one sort or another have been used for this purpose. The use of strong salt solution — brine — to preserve foods from putrefaction, that is to say, bacterial decomposition, has gone on for centuries. The curing of bacon, and the pickling of pork and other foods are additional examples. Salt, oils, vinegar and wine have all been used in the treatment of wounds to prevent or cure sepsis.

At first, the chemical substances used were crude substances easily available for everyday purposes, whose value as disinfectants was quite incidental to their ordinary use. As the science of chemistry slowly developed, simple chemicals such as mineral acids and alkalis — vitriol, soda and potash — came to be used for disinfection as did solutions of the salts of various heavy metals such as silver and mercury salts. These substances were relatively cheap, but had serious disadvantages. The chief of these were that they were corrosive and dangerous to human tissues and could not be handled safely without careful precautions. Moreover, they were liable to damage clothing, dressings and instruments. These disadvantages were overcome to some extent by diluting the substances; however, the more they were diluted, the less effective they became as disinfectants.

In the middle of the last century a great advance in the chemical industry led to a revolution in the use of chemical disinfectants. This was the discovery of the fractional distillation of coal. From this process, numerous chemical substances suddenly became available very cheaply. Among these was carbolic acid or phenol, which had already been known to be an effective and useful disinfectant, and still is widely used in various mixtures which are mentioned below.

Carbolic acid was much used by Lister when he started the practice of antiseptic surgery, a practice which completely altered the prospects for the rapid recovery of patients in surgical wards.

Many other disinfectants are produced by the distillation of coal-tar. All the phenolic disinfectants in use today, such as the 'white fluids' and 'black fluids', are coal-tar derivatives. 'Lysol' is a mixture of cresol, a phenol compound, with soaps. The aniline dyes, such as flavine and gentian violet, are also coal-tar derivatives, as are the chloroxylenol compounds such as 'dettol' and chlorhexidine ('hibitane').

In recent years, the increasing development of the chemical industry has led to the introduction of large numbers of new and excellent chemical disinfectants and antiseptics. In fact, such a bewildering variety of chemicals are now available that it is as well to look rather hard at the purposes of chemical sterilisation.

Quite apart from chemicals, there are many ways of preventing the appearance of microbes in dangerous numbers. Generally speaking, disinfection by heat or irradiation is preferable to using chemicals whenever this is practicable. It does not involve the introduction of foreign chemical substances of which harmful traces may have to be washed away.

Disinfection would be more effective if the following questions were asked (and answered) whenever the use of a chemical disinfectant were contemplated:

1. What exactly is the purpose of disinfection in this particular case? Is not simple cleaning with soap and water all that is required?

2. What are the effective and safe chemical substances to do the particular job, and what is the correct concentration?

3. Which is the best (that is, the most effective and safest) method of applying the solution?

4. Are any special safety measures necessary (for example, wearing rubber gloves)?

5. Are there likely to be any undesirable after-effects? or residual effects? Should the disinfectant be washed off afterwards?

In this section we are not considering the use of bacterial agents to kill or prevent the growth of bacteria inside the body. Antibiotics and chemotherapeutic drugs are usually used for this purpose, and are considered in Chapter 8.

Chemical disinfectants should be used only when heat treatment or irradiation is not practicable. For example, chemicals should not be used to sterilise dressings or instruments when it is possible to sterilise these with heat treatment, as it usually is.

The following are the most important reasons for using chemical disinfectants:

1. To cleanse the skin: It is not possible to sterilise the skin by using disinfectants, but the number of microbes on the surface of the skin may be reduced (see page 123).

2. On wound dressings, to prevent contamination and remove sepsis.

3. To treat sites, such as the nose, from which microbes may be broadcast, and hence reduce cross-infection.

4. To sterilise objects, such as trolleys, which come into contact with sterile instruments or dressings.

5. To disinfect objects such as baths, bowls, tables, chairs, lockers, and so on.

6. To sterilise walls, floors, and ceilings in operating theatres and elsewhere in hospitals.

7. For sanitary purposes, to disinfect drains, etc.

Some general principles about the use of chemical disinfectants should be borne in mind; these are largely common sense which is a good guide to the use of chemical disinfectants.

(a) The activity of many chemical disinfectants is reduced by the presence of traces of organic matter, e.g. dirt or pus.

(b) When used in concentrations which are not toxic to human beings (e.g. on the skin or on dressings) chemical disinfectants are not usually effective in killing spores of tetanus or gas gangrene.

(c) The action of chemical disinfectants on microbes is not instantaneous. Over a wide range, the number of bacteria killed depends on:

(1) Concentration of disinfectant.

(2) Time of exposure.

(3) Temperature.

In other words, chemical disinfection will be more effective the more concentrated the disinfectant, the longer the microbes are left in contact with it, and the hotter the solution.

One often sees surgeons and nurses putting their hands into a bowl of disinfectant solution, and taking them out almost immediately. This momentary exposure is not likely to kill many bacteria, unless the concentration of disinfectant is quite high. The hands should be left exposed for an appreciable time for the sterilisation to be effective.

Similarly, people have been known to pour a spoonful of disinfectant into a bath of water before getting into it, in the hope that by doing this they are sterilising the bath water. This is a vain hope. To sterilise a bath of moderate size in a short time, much larger quantities, possibly several pints, of disinfectant would be needed.

(d) Some disinfectants kill some microbes more easily than others. For example, gentian violet kills staphylococci easily in concentrations of 1/1,000 in water. However, it does not always kill streptococci at this concentration.

Many chemical disinfectants, particularly the old-fashioned ones, are corrosive and harmful when in contact with the skin and tissues of human beings. As the chemical industry has developed, disinfectants have become more and more selective in their action against microbes, and more and more bland and harmless to human beings. One can conceive of the ideal disinfectant as one which kills all microbes readily but has no harmful action of any sort on human tissues or on fabrics. This ideal will never be quite attained, any more than any other ideals. However, we are not far from it today.

The Use of Chemical Disinfectants in Hospitals

The emphasis should always be on cleanliness, and on the removal of microbes incidental to this, rather than on killing microbes as an end in itself. Washing removes dirt, and dirt contains microbes: 'Take good care of the dirt and the germs will take care of themselves'.

The use of disinfectants for various purposes in hospitals is best decided by a small group of experts, including senior nurses, the bacteriologist, and the pharmacist. Clear instructions should be prepared and should be issued to the wards and departments.

Much time, trouble and confusion can be saved if the number of different disinfectant solutions used in a hospital is kept to a minimum. Most jobs can be done by a single standard solution, which can be issued in bulk by the dispensary.

Review of Chemical Disinfectants

The following review deals with some of the main types of disinfectant. It is impossible to mention all chemical disinfectants, or even all types, as there are so many. The ones dealt with here are those which are most widely used. They are grouped in alphabetical order, as follows:

1. Alcohol and Ether.
2. Aniline dyes.

3. Chlorhexidine and hexachlorophane.
4. Ethylene oxide.
5. Formaldehyde.
6. Glutaraldehyde.
7. Halogens, iodophors, hypochlorites.
8. Heavy metals.
9. Oxidising agents.
10. Phenolics, including chloroxylenols.
11. Quaternary ammonium compounds.

Concentrations to be used: It is not possible to give dogmatic guidance as to the concentrations which should be used of many of the disinfectants. These depend on the particular preparation used or the strength of the stock solution dispensed. However, in the case of stock solutions, **clear instructions about concentrations should be given on each stock bottle. In every ward and department where disinfectants are used, a chart giving clear instructions about concentrations should be in some conspicuous place.**

1. Alcohol and Ether

Ethyl alcohol and **methylated spirit** by itself is quite a useful disinfectant, and it is most effective at a concentration of 70%. It has the big disadvantage of stinging raw and broken skin surfaces, the scrotum, and mucous membranes, so it should never be used on these surfaces in a conscious patient. It is best used as a solvent for some other disinfectant e.g. flavine or another dye, or a quaternary ammonium salt.

    Ether is not a disinfectant; few microbes are killed by it. It is, however, a very useful fat solvent. Ether evaporates very rapidly at ordinary room temperatures, withdrawing heat from the skin as it does so and hence making the skin feel cold.

2. Aniline Dyes e.g. flavine, acriflavine, proflavine, gentian violet, brilliant green

These are all derived from the chemical aniline, which is related to phenol or carbolic acid. They are moderately effective disinfectants, and may be used for sterilising the skin in 1/1000 strength in 70% alcohol. If used for raw surfaces or mucous membranes, watery solution should, of course, be used since alcoholic solutions sting.

Advantages

    (a) Some have a slight astingent action e.g. gentian violet.
    (b) Cheap.

Disadvantages

1/1000 gentian violet has been much used in the past for treating mucous surfaces for thrush, a fungus disease. In this form it has been used in the mouth and in the vagina. However, its intense staining properties have made it unpopular; it stains clothes and bedclothes indelibly. It has now been almost completely replaced by Nystatin and other antifungal antibiotics.

3. Chlorhexidine and Hexachlorophane

Chlorhexidine ('Hibitane') is a white powder which is bacteriostatic and bactericidal against a wide range of microbes. It is of low toxicity, and is quite safe to use on the skin and mucous membranes. It is used in handcreams and nasal creams to kill staphylococci and cure staphylococcal carriers; in nasal creams it is sometimes mixed with an antibiotic such as neomycin. Solutions of chlorhexidine are also used for pre-operative sterilisation, in concentrations of 1/5000 (or 1/250 'Hibitane concentrate').

Advantages

    (a) Colourless.
    (b) Soluble.
    (c) Relatively non-toxic.

Disadvantages

Not very active against *Proteus* and *Ps. aeruginosa.*
    Hexochlorophane has been much used in the past but is restricted in some countries owing to possible danger to small infants. It is compounded into soaps and into complex detergents such as 'Phisohex' for pre-operative scrubbing up and general handwashing. 'Phisohex' is said to act by removing the surface microbes and forming a protective film on the skin which prevents the deeper microbes from reaching the surface.

Advantages

Colourless.

Disadvantages

    (a) Low solubility in water.
    (b) Not very active against *Proteus* and *Ps. pyocyanea.*

4. Ethylene Oxide

A gas used for sterilising large objects of surgical equipment.

Advantages

High penetration.

Disadvantages

  (a) Very explosive.
  (b) Irritant.
  (c) Volatile.

5. Formaldehyde

This is a gas at ordinary temperatures, and is used for sterilising rooms. Solutions are also effective disinfectants. 'Formalin' is 40% solution of formaldehyde in water.

Advantages

  (a) Effective spore-killer.
  (b) Cheap.

Disadvantages

  (a) Pungent smell.
  (b) Irritating to the tissues.
  (c) Poor penetration.

6. Glutaraldehyde

A liquid disinfectant, often used at 2% strength. Solutions remain active for 2 weeks after preparation.

Advantages

  (a) Wide range of action, including spore-bearing organisms, tubercle bacilli and viruses.
  (b) Does not damage endoscopic instruments, or plastics, rubber, or the markings on thermometers.

Disadvantages

Very irritant to the eye, slightly irritant to skin and mucous-membranes.

7. Halogens — Iodine and chlorine

Iodine is used as tincture of iodine, a solution of iodine with potassium iodide in alcohol. It is quite a good skin disinfectant, and stains the skin brown.

Advantages

Colour — sometimes an advantage in marking out operation sites.

Disadvantages

(a) Many people are sensitive to iodine, and its use on the skin may provoke allergic reactions in the form of urticaria, conjunctivitis, etc. Patients should *always* be tested for allergy by a skin test before iodine is used on them.

(b) Inactivation by organic material; while it disinfects intact skin, it is not much use once an incision has been made, and there is blood in the vicinity.

(c) 'Stings' raw and broken skin, mucous surfaces, and the scrotum, as does any alcoholic solution.

(d) Stains fabric dark blue, and this stain cannot be removed without chemical treatment.

There seems to be little use today for iodine; more modern disinfectants can do the same job equally well, without any of the disadvantages.

Iodophors such as 'betadine', are solutions which contain iodine but are much less irritant, and do not stain the skin. They are said to be equally effective.

Chlorine is a gas slightly soluble in water, and is a powerful disinfectant. Its solubility has led to its use as a means of sterilising water. Piped water supplies are sometimes 'chlorinated', and so are swimming baths. However, chlorine is irritant and if too much is put into a swimming bath, the bathers' eyes may become inflamed.

Hypochlorites, e.g. Eusol, 'Milton', Dakins' fluid

These are very useful general disinfectants. They are alkaline solutions containing chlorine from which the chlorine is easily liberated, exerting a disinfectant effect. The alkali in the solution enables it to dissolve organic matter such as pus and mucus. Hypochlorites are therefore very useful for dressing infected areas such as discharging abscesses and wounds, and for irrigating these. They are also used in nurseries for keeping babies' feeding bottles and teats sterile. However, the solutions used for this purpose should be changed frequently, at least every day.

Hypochlorites can also be used for disinfecting large objects of equipment and the surfaces of furniture.

The concentration at which they are used depends on the preparation dispensed.

Advantages

(a) Colourless.

(b) Wide range of activity, probably including the virus of serum hepatitis.

(c) Cheap.

Disadvantages

(a) Smell.
(b) Solution needs to be changed frequently.
There are many modern organic disinfectants which liberate chlorine and act in the same way as hypochlorites, e.g. Chloramine-T.

8. Heavy Metals

Biniodide and **perchloride of mercury; silver nitrate.**

These substances have been used for many years. In the concentrated state they are dangerously corrosive, but they are safe when used in high dilutions, e.g. 1/1000. In these solutions they are not disinfectant but bacteriostatic.

Advantages

(a) Effective sterilisers for skin or body surface.
(b) Cheap.

Disadvantages

Very easily inactivated by traces of organic matter such as dirt or pus.

Organic Mercurials are used to disinfect body surfaces, e.g.

> Thiomersal (merthiolate)
> Mercurochrome
> Phenylmercuric nitrate
> Nitromersal

Advantages

(a) Relatively harmless.
(b) Useful as preservatives. Thus, phenylmercuric nitrate can be used to preserve solutions, such as eyedrops.

Disadvantages

Bacteriostatic.

9. Oxidising Agents

Potassium permanganate. This salt forms a mauve solution in water, which is a moderately powerful disinfectant and has some astringent action. It is therefore of value in treating discharging septic lesions, which it helps to dry up.

Advantages

(a) Slight astringent action.
(b) Cheap.

Disadvantages

(a) Easily inactivated by organic material.
(b) Stains many things brown, for example, it stains teeth brown if it is used in a mouthwash.

Peroxide of Hydrogen is a weak disinfectant which bubbles up when poured out. This makes it useful for irrigating deep wounds and sinuses; sometimes the bubbles may lift out fragments of pus and debris from such lesions.

10. **Phenolics**

Probably the most commonly used disinfectants today are derivatives of phenol. There is a large number of phenolic disinfectants which range from crude and dangerously corrosive substances such as phenol itself (carbolic acid), and lysol, to refined and relatively harmless compounds such as chlorhexidine (hibitane) and hexachlorophane, which have already been mentioned.

Phenol and cresol mixtures, such as 'lysol', 'sudol', and various 'black fluids' and 'white fluids', are used for large scale, sanitary type disinfection of drains, floors, and so on.

On floors they should be used in about 1/160 strength. They may be used for washing out baths, and washing down trolleys in the same strength.

Advantages

(a) Effective against all types of vegetative microbes and, given several hours exposure time, against spore-bearers.
(b) Cheap.

Disadvantages

(a) Dangerous to use. In concentrated form, they damage the skin and produce burns on the skin in sensitive people even when used diluted. Rubber gloves should be used when these substances are handled; **they should never be allowed to come into contact with the skin, even when diluted.**
(b) Messy. Much water has to be used to get rid of them, and it is difficult to remove the last traces.
(c) Pungent, persistent and characteristic smell. Some people like this,

but nowadays most find it has unpleasant, 'institutional' associations.

There are many mixtures of synthetic phenolic disinfectants available today which can do the same disinfecting job as well as the crude phenolics without all of the disadvantages, though they must be handled with care.

An example is 'Clearsol', which is a derivative of phenol which is not so toxic or corrosive as the substances mentioned above. It can be used for most sterilising purposes in the ward, apart from those involving contact with the skin of patients. 'Tego' is a mixture containing detergents and phenolics which is also safe and effective; it is much used in hospitals.

Chloroxylenol is the name of a substance chemically derived from phenol which forms the basis of a large number of modern proprietary disinfectants, such as 'Dettol', etc. Different brands differ in their exact composition, and in the other substances which are mixed with the chloroxylenol. The concentration of the solution is also varied from time to time.

Most of these substances are sold in the form of yellow, clear, rather syrupy liquids, which form a white, milky emulsion with a characteristically pungent smell when mixed with water. The concentration at which they should be used depends on the particular preparation.

Advantages

(a) Comparatively harmless even in high concentrations. Even if used undiluted on the skin they will not harm most people provided they are washed off quickly.

(b) Most people like the smell.

Disadvantages

(a) Rather high concentrations are necessary, anything from 100% to 10%.

(b) Expensive.

11. Quaternary Ammonium Compounds

There are many of these, including **benzalkonium** (Roccal; Zephiran); **cetrimide** (Cetavlon); **domiphen** (Bradosol); **laurolinium** (Laurodin) and **dequalinium** (Dequadin). They are widely used in watery or alcoholic solutions for cleansing the skin (see below) on surgical dressings, and for general disinfection. They are also used in creams, ointments and sprays.

They are effective in 1% strength, or even less, against many types of microbes. However, the concentration to be used depends on the particular preparation.

Advantages

(a) Colourless.

(b) Relatively non-toxic.

Disadvantages

(a) Selective in their action. Some bacteria, e.g. *Ps. aeruginosa* or tubercle bacilli, are hardly affected by them.

(b) Expensive.

(c) Many people do not like cetrimide because it is slippery to the touch.

Some Special Problems

Disinfecting the Skin

The bacteria which live on the skin may be divided into two groups. There are the 'transient' flora which are temporarily deposited on the skin, and are on the whole easily removed by washing with soap and water or disinfectant solutions. These often include pathogenic organisms such as *E. coli, Staph. aureus* and *Ps. aeruginosa.*

The 'resident' flora live and multiply on the skin, usually in crevices or in hair follicles and sweat glands. Any movement of the skin may push them up to the surface. These organisms are usually harmless, but they may include *Staph. aureus.* They cannot be completely removed by washing or scrubbing. Attempts to sterilise the skin cannot, therefore, be fully effective. None the less, it is possible to reduce the resident flora of the hands of surgeons and nurses quite a lot by the use of various disinfectants, some of which have a cumulative effect if used over a long period.

Treatment of Operation Sites

The skin flora can be much reduced by a single treatment with 5% laurolinium, 0.5% chlorhexidine in alcohol, tincture of iodine, or many other substances. Repeated treatment for two or three days before operation will reduce the flora still more.

The Nose

The nasal mucous membrane is the most important source of *Staphylococcus aureus.* 50% of nurses carry it at any one time, and nasal carriage is widespread among the general population, who become patients in hospital wards. It is important to try to reduce or prevent the carriage of staphylococci in nurses on surgical wards and other wards where there are patients at special risk. Antiseptic ointments and sprays are used for this purpose. These may contain 'Soframycin' (framycetin with gramicidin), 'Naseptin' (chlorhexidine and neomycin) or other mixtures.

In the Wards

So far as ward objects such as tables, trolleys and lockers are concerned, the best way to keep down the numbers of microbes is to maintain a high standard of general cleanliness. Chemical disinfectants should be used in addition to soap and water for a greater effect.

Instruments

It is a dangerous mistake to imagine that instruments can be effectively sterilised with chemicals. Chemical disinfection is never the best way of sterilising instruments or apparatus, because the chemical must always be washed away with a good deal of water. Even if 'sterile water' is used, this introduces the danger of contamination.

Wherever possible, instruments should be autoclaved, ovened, or sterilised by irradiation.

Respiratory and Anaesthetic Apparatus

Ventilators, respirators, incubators, and anaesthetic machines are often difficult to disinfect. Removable parts can sometimes be sterilised by autoclaving, but one must be careful that fine mechanical components will stand up to this without damage. Sometimes the whole apparatus can be put into a tent or bag and sterilised with a disinfectant vapour such as ethylene oxide or formaldehyde. Other methods are running a chemical disinfectant solution through the apparatus, or discharging into it a disinfectant vapour such as formaldehyde. Before the apparatus is used again, it is most important to ensure that there are no toxic or irritant traces of the disinfectant.

Sterile Water

The only acceptable sterile water is water which has been autoclaved after being bottled, in sealed bottles. No fluid in a bottle with an ordinary bark cork should ever be regarded as sterile, since it is impossible to sterilise such corks. Rubber bungs, on the other hand, can be sterilised by boiling or autoclaving. Again, bottles of sterile water should only be regarded as sterile when they are intact. Once they have been opened, they are no longer sterile. This means that a bottle of sterile water should never be used more than once. Bowls of so-called 'sterile water' left open to the air are a dangerous source of infection in operating theatres.

The same applies, of course, to sterile saline.

CHAPTER 10

RESISTANCE TO INFECTION:
AN INTRODUCTION TO IMMUNITY

Everybody knows the meaning of the word 'immunity'; it is the power of the individual to resist disease. This is a complicated subject, for there are many factors involved in immunity, and not all of them are full understood. Much of it is outside the scope of this book, and what follows is an attempt to give a simplified picture.

The word 'immunity' is also used nowadays in a narrower sense as a technical term to denote the operation in the body of some of the mechanisms which make for resistance. For example, we talk about 'auto-immune diseases', and about Rhesus-negative mothers being 'immunised' against the red cells of their infants. This double use of the word occasionally leads to some confusion.

While the subject is complicated, it is one which most people today know something about. Everyone knows that attacks of many types of infectious disease, such as measles, leave one immune against further attacks, so that a second attack is unlikely and unusual. Everyond knows too that it is possible to immunise people artificially against many diseases, for example, measles and diphtheria. It is also a matter of common observation that some people are more resistant to disease than others. Some never seem to know a day's illness whereas others always seem to be getting coughs and colds in the winter.

Perhaps the best way to understand the mechanisms of immunity to infection is to consider them systematically, and the following table is a convenient scheme:

Immunity:　(a) Innate — Species; Individual.
　　　　　　 (b) Acquired — Natural — active
　　　　　　　　　　　　　　　　　　 — passive;
　　　　　　　　　　　　 Artificial — active
　　　　　　　　　　　　　　　　　　 — passive.

Innate Immunity

By this is meant immunity which is inherent in an individual irrespective of environmental factors.

Species immunity. A degree of immunity is inherent in each animal species, or, in other words, some species of animals do not get the diseases which others get. Thus, human beings do not contract distemper of dogs, or foot-and-mouth disease of cattle, except as an extremely rare occurrence. They are immune to these diseases. Similarly, dogs and cattle do not get measles or poliomyelitis, which are diseases of human beings.

This is what is meant by species immunity. Some microbes cause a serious disease in one animal species but a mild disease in another. Thus, *Salmonella typhimurium* is a bacterium which causes a serious and often fatal disease in mice, 'mouse typhoid'. In human beings it causes bacterial food-poisoning and is in fact the commonest cause of this, a troublesome but mild disease.

It is often stated that different 'races' of humanity have different immunity to different diseases. These statements are based on such observations as that immigrants to this country seem to develop tuberculosis more often than English people. Another example is that remote communities, once brought into contact with civilisation, suffer serious outbreaks of such diseases as measles which do not affect our own society anything like so severely. While such things as this undoubtedly happen, they are due to environmental factors such as differences in living standards or the degree of exposure of members of the community to the infection.

For example, housing conditions, and the presence or absence of overcrowding, can affect resistance to disease. Nutrition is another factor; the majority of the world's population are inadequately nourished and are more liable to infective disease on this account than is the well-nourished minority. Another is the lack of opportunity of many isolated communities of coming into contact with a particular microbe, and hence of developing resistance to it. When people from these communities migrate to more populous areas, they often go down with an infection which they are meeting for the first time.

Sometimes several of these factors can be seen to operate together to diminish resistance. Thus, immigrants into this country often live in poor conditions in crowded lodging houses, and do not get enough to eat, and so on; all these conditions would increase their likelihood to develop tuberculosis quite apart from any innate difference in resistance.

There is no real evidence that there are any differences of immunity between different human groups other than can be accounted for by such environmental factors. In any case, human 'races' are now so mixed up that any innate differences which might once have existed are likely to have been ironed out.

Individual immunity. Differences between individuals can well affect immunity. If two communities of children are considered, let us say a community of well-off children in a private school, and a community of children of similar age in a depressed area suffering from unemployment, the latter will show a higher incidence of many diseases than the former. Respiratory illnesses and rheumatic fever are examples.

Tuberculosis is another good example of a disease whose incidence is clearly related to standards of living. Others are the great epidemic scourges such as typhus, cholera, and plague. These all occur most commonly where living conditions are at their worst and where people are most crowded together, as they are in the great cities of the East such as Calcutta and Dacca.

Variations in the life of a particular individual such as the state of nutrition, fatigue, indulgence in alcohol, and smoking, can also affect his or her susceptibility to disease. Some factors such as the intake of Vitamin A have a specific effect in increasing resistance to infection.

Fatigue almost certainly affects resistance. Overwork predisposes to tuberculosis, and muscular activity undoubtedly affects the outcome of infection by polio virus; it may make all the difference between an abortive attack without paralysis and a severe or even fatal paralytic attack. It is a common observation, too, that in winter a 'run-down' overworked state makes a cold or an attack of flu more likely. Hot meals in winter have a definite psychological value, which may well improve resistance to winter ailments such as the common cold. Over-indulgence in alcohol also appears to increase susceptibility to tuberculosis and venereal disease.

Smoking damages the respiratory mucous membrane and increases its susceptibility to respiratory infections, quite apart from its effect on the incidence of cancer of the lung.

There are many individual defence mechanisms that protect against infection.

The **skin** is an effective barrier which has definite bactericidal properties. If suspensions of living microbes, apart from those which normally live on the skin, are painted on it with a swab or a brush, many will be killed in an hour or two by contact with the epidermis. This effect is due to the acid reaction of the skin. On the other hand, broken or grazed or burned skin is a common portal of entry of microbes, as is macerated skin, that is, skin damaged by excessive moisture. Areas which are often moist are most likely to become infected; such as the skin in the flexures of the body—the axillae, underneath the breasts of a woman, the groins, the umbilicus, and between the toes. So are those areas with an allergic or eczematous rash. The resistance to infection of the skin depends on its being healthy and intact (see Chapter 3).

The **eyes** are particularly resistant to infection, largely because of **lysozyme**, a powerful bactericide present in tears, which are themselves the secretion of the lacrimal glands.

The acid secretion of the **stomach** protects against food-borne infection; the greater the gastric acidity, the higher the protection. This is illustrated by resistance to cholera. The cholera bacillus is easily killed by acid, and people with a high gastric acidity escape the disease altogether during an epidemic. On the other hand, people with low acidity are particularly susceptible to cholera.

The **vagina**, in the adult, has an acid wall which discourages the growth of foreign bacteria and acts to some extent as a barrier against infection.

The **blood serum** contains chemical substances, such as **complement** and **properdin**, which are bactericidal. One of the constituents of the serum proteins is called **gamma globulin** (IgG); in the normal individual this contains antibodies against a number of microbes. A very small number of people have no gamma globulin in the blood; this is a disease called **agamma-globulinemia**. They are abnormally susceptible to infections and are always getting ill.

The white cells of the blood are another important defence against infection. The main function of the polymorph leucocytes is to ingest and kill invading bacteria, and this action is most marked in **pyogenic** infections. Pus consists largely of accumulations of polymorph leucocytes and the bacteria against whose invasion they are fighting. If the white blood cells of an individual are reduced or absent, as happens in the rare disease **agranulocytosis**, his capacity to resist infection is very seriously impaired. Patients with this disease may become ill owing to invasion by microbes which would be harmless in the normal person. Overwhelming infection is the chief danger to life in agranulocytosis, and must be guarded against.

These are some of the mechanisms which in the healthy person safeguard the body against disease. They provide, of course, only relative protection, which can be broken down.

Natural Acquired Immunity

It is well known that immunity can be acquired during life, without artificial immunisation. The small infant is susceptible to most infections; as he or she gets older he develops immunity to some, often as a result of contracting and recovering from the disease.

All acquired immunity is due to the acquisition of **antibodies**. These are chemical substances manufactured by cells called *B-lymphocytes*. They react with and neutralise substances called **antigens** which are present in microbes, and which are responsible for the microbes' power to produce disease. This neutralisation process renders the microbes innocuous. Hence the action of antibodies is to protect against their harmful effects. The production of antibodies is stimulated by infection, which introduces the microbial antigen into the body. Here is an example of how the process works:

A person who has no immunity to a particular microbe becomes infected with it. If the infection is a heavy one, he may become ill of the disease caused by the microbe.

If it is a light one, he will not become ill. In either event, however, his body, stimulated by the presence of the foreign microbe and its antigens, starts to produce antibodies against it some days after the beginning of the infection. These antibodies get into the bloodstream and body tissues, and when they meet the microbe they neutralise it, rendering it harmless.

If the person is ill of the disease, the development of antibodies will improve his condition and may bring the illness to an end, unless the infection is an overwhelming one. Sometimes the outcome is touch and go between the natural defences of the body, including the antibodies, and the disease-producing mechanisms, appropriately called the **aggressive mechanisms**, of the microbe.

Whether the result of the infection is a definite disease ('clinical infection') or, in the case of light infection, no appreciable disease ('sub-clinical infection'), the individual, if he survives, is left with the power to produce antibodies in the future. So he is left with an immunity against the particular microbe.

Antigens are substances in microbes which stimulate the production of antibodies. Most microbes contain not one but many antigens, and hence give rise to the production of not one but many antibodies. So the result of an infection is often the development of a number of antibodies by the host, which together produce immunity against a particular microbe. Some microbes have antigens in common. For example, one microbe, let us say the typhoid bacillus, may contain antigens which we may call A, B, C, D, E. Infection with the typhoid bacillus will result in the patient developing antibodies against A, B, C, D, E, and hence, if he recovers from the infection, he will be immune to typhoid in the future. But another enteric type of organism may have antigens B, C, D, E, F. Infection with typhoid will result in a high degree of immunity against this organism too, because the patient will have antibodies B, C, D, E which will protect him against the corresponding antigens in the second organisms (Fig. 33).

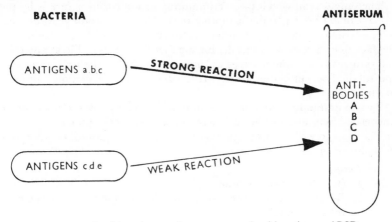

Fig. 33. Bacteria with antigens a, b, c react strongly with antiserum ABCD.
Bacteria with antigens c, d, e react less strongly

Some antigens, for example those of the typhoid bacillus, are actually part of the structure of the bacterial body, and cannot be separated from it without breaking up the bacterium. Other antigens can easily be separated from the bacterium. Such are the exotoxins of diphtheria and tetanus, which are soluble substances excreted by the organisms.

This is a simplified picture of the mechanism of acquired immunity, which operates in all types of infection. This view still leaves many questions unanswered. For example, there are many diseases, such as measles, typhoid and whooping cough, in which a first attack brings a good deal of immunity and second attacks are rare. There are others, such as the common cold and influenza, in which repeated attacks occur. What is the explanation of this?

There are several explanations, all of which fit in with the above picture. In the case of influenza, it is that the viruses are constantly undergoing slight change, by natural selection and mutation. So each new outbreak is due to a virus which is antigenically, that is to say chemically, slightly different from those which caused the previous outbreak. So immunity conferred against a particular outbreak will not protect fully, and may not protect at all, against the virus causing a later outbreak.

So far as colds are concerned, it is now known that there are many different viruses which may cause the disease. Any particular attack of a cold will bring immunity against the virus that caused it, but not necessarily against other cold viruses which may also be prevalent and therefore cause a second cold a short time after the first.

So far, the discussion has been about acquired immunity, in which the person makes his own antibodies in response to a stimulus from outside. This is therefore called **active immunity**. There is a different way of acquiring immunity, in which antibodies manufactured by some other person or animal enter the body. This is called **passive immunity**.

The only way in which passive immunity can occur in nature is by the passage of antibodies from the mother to the foetus across the placenta, or, as may also happen, in the mothers' colostrum or milk. This accounts for the fact that the newborn infant, for the first few weeks of life at any rate, is immune to the same diseases as those to which the mother is immune; the infant has antibodies which have entered his circulation from the mother.

Passive immunity may also be acquired artificially, by the injection of antiserum from another human being or a laboratory animal.

The ways in which immunity may be naturally acquired may therefore be summed up as follows:

 (a) Active.
  1. By subclinical infection.
  2. By an attack of the disease, or of a disease due to an antigenically related microbe.
 (b) Passive.
  By transfer of antibodies from the mother, usually across the placenta, but possibly also in the colostrum or milk.

Artificially Acquired Immunity

Doctors are constantly being called upon to protect people, especially children, against the possibility of their developing particular types of infectious disease; in other words to immunise them. The development of methods of immunity over the past fifty years or so is one of the greatest advances in medicine, and has probably saved more lives than any other, except possibly the development of antibiotics. The best example of this is the immunisation campaign against diphtheria, which has brought about the almost total disappearance of this disease from Great Britain, as mentioned on page 53. Thousands of children's lives are saved every year by diphtheria immunisation.

Many other striking examples can be quoted. The abolition of smallpox as an endemic disease is largely due to vaccination. One of the reasons for the great reduction of the incidence of tuberculosis in Great Britain is that immunisation by a vaccine, BCG, is now made available to all school-children and is widely practised.

The effectiveness of vaccination campaigns is well shown in wartime, when thousands of servicemen and women are sent to countries such as Africa and India where sanitary standards are low and infectious disease is rife. All service personnel are immunised against smallpox, typhoid and paratyphoid; they may also be immunised against cholera. As a result, the incidence of these diseases in service men and women is very low.

Another example of how immunisation may reduce the incidence of a disease to a rarity is that of poliomyelitis. Until immunisation became possible a few years ago, several thousands of cases occurred every year in Great Britain, with many deaths. In the last few years the figures in this country have been very low indeed, and show no sign of increasing again.

Methods of Producing Artificial Active Immunity

Most artificial immunisation is active immunisation, that is, the patient is given the antigenic stimulus to produce his own antibodies. There are various ways of doing this which depend on the particular disease against which one is immunising. A number of different vaccines may also be combined in a single preparation, as in 'triple vaccine' containing diphtheria toxoid, tetanus toxoid, and whooping cough vaccine. The use of such preparations reduces the number of injections which have to be given to children. Combined vaccines are just as effective as single ones.

1. By administration of a toxin or toxoid

Some bacteria produce a toxin, or poison, which diffuses into the medium in which the organism is grown and can be separated from the microbe and purified. The diphtheria and tetanus bacilli are the best examples of this. In the living body, it is the toxin, circulating in the patient, that is responsible for the disease. If the toxin is neutralised by antibody, which is called antitoxin, the patient will easily overcome the infection.

Active immunisation in this case consists of giving the person injections of a substance which will stimulate him to produce antitoxin. Of course, one does not use toxin for this purpose. If this were used, it would have a poisonous effect on the individual and would be almost as bad as the disease itself. Fortunately, it is possible to alter toxin slightly by chemical treatment, producing a substance called **toxoid** which is just as effective antigenically as toxin, but has no harmful effects. That is to say, injections of toxoid are effective in stimulating the production of antitoxin.

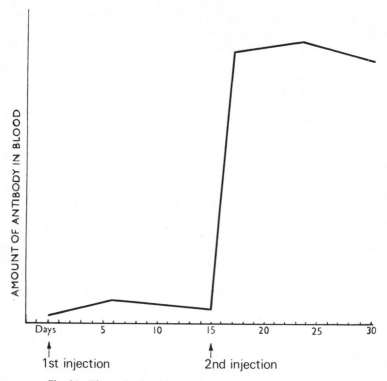

Fig. 34. The antibody response after the first and second doses of
a non-living antigen

In active immunisation against diphtheria and tetanus, it is necessary to give more than one injection of toxoid.

A single injection of a non-living substance such as toxoid is usually insufficient stimulus to the body for it to produce much antibody. The first injection sensitises the individual; it causes his cells to alter in such a way that they will produce antibody when they receive a second injection. This **sensitisation** process takes a few weeks. Four weeks after the first injection of toxoid, a second injection is given; this causes a rapid production of antitoxin which circulates in the bloodstream and neutralises any toxin formed by the pathogenic organisms should they enter the body at any time. The interval between the injections need not be exactly four weeks, though this is the period which gives the best results. Anything over two weeks will do. Less than two weeks will not do, and a second injection given so soon after the first will not be effective. It takes at least this length of time to sensitise the antibody-forming tissues, that is, to train them to produce antibody.

A third injection of toxoid, after another interval of four weeks or more, raises the antitoxin level still further.

This process is illustrated in Figure 34.

After a course of immunisation, which usually consists of three injections, the level of circulating antibody gradually declines, and after some years it may fall to almost nothing. However, once the body has been sensitised it retains the capacity to produce antibody again after any antigenic stimulus. So that if, years later, it is necessary to restore a high level of immunity, this can be done rapidly by a single injection of antigen. It is usual to give a 'booster dose', as it is called, of diphtheria toxoid to children at about the age of five years, to reinforce their 'primary' immunity which is generally given in the first year of life.

A large number of patients in hospital casualty departments are people with dirty wounds who may have to be protected against tetanus. If they have previously been given active immunisation against tetanus, all that is needed is for them to have a booster dose of tetanus toxoid, which will restore their immunity to a high level. This is, of course, in addition to the necessary surgical treatment of the wound and is not a substitute for it.

2. By administration of killed organisms

Many bacteria do not produce exotoxins; nor do viruses. Active immunisation against these organisms takes the form of administration of the microbe itself, either killed or in an altered form. Killed vaccines are used in immunisation against whooping cough, typhoid and paratyphoid fevers, influenza, and cholera. The Salk type of polio vaccine is another example of a killed vaccine.

Such vaccines, like toxoids, have to be given more than once to produce lasting immunity; three injections at monthly intervals are the most effective way of administering them.

It is important that the killed microbe is given in a potent form, one in which the majority of the antigens are preserved so that full immunity can be produced. The method of growing the microbes and of killing them is very important, and profoundly influences the effectiveness of a vaccine.

Many killed vaccines are harmless. However, some of them may give rise to reactions.

Typhoid-paratyphoid vaccines (TAB) quite often cause pain and stiffness of the limb in which they are injected, accompanied by fever and malaise. This illness lasts about 24 hours, and it is important to warn patients that they may be unwell for a day or so after a TAB vaccination.

The polio vaccines are a mixture of various strains of each of the three main types of polio virus.

3. By administration of living microbes

Some killed microbes are ineffective as vaccines because the injection of the killed organisms does not give rise to the production of protective antibodies. To produce immunity, the microbes have to be introduced alive into the body, so that they can multiply there for a time. The only effective vaccines against the diseases which these microbes cause must consist of **living organisms**.

The use of living organisms for vaccines immediately raises obvious difficulties, of which the chief is that there is a danger that the live organisms will give rise to the disease which they are intended to prevent. Obviously one cannot safely inject or administer the unchanged virulent organism. There are various ways of getting over this. One is by using **attenuated** organisms, that is to say, microbes which have been artificially weakened so that they are not capable of causing disease, though they give rise to the same antibodies, when injected, as do the fully virulent microbes. An example of this is the use of BCG vaccine for immunisation against tuberculosis. BCG, as mentioned in Chapter 5, is a strain of tubercle bacillus which has been attenuated for many years by growing it on an artificial culture medium in the laboratory. It is incapable of producing serious or fatal progressive disease like the fully virulent tubercle bacillus; it produces a small abscess in the skin when it is injected intradermally.

Another example is the use of oral 'Sabin' vaccine to immunise against polio. The oral vaccines are an alternative and probably more effective method than the use of killed vaccines which have already been mentioned. They consist of a mixture of various types of attenuated polio virus. When swallowed, they multiply in the gut, but do not enter the bloodstream. None the less, they give rise to antibodies against virulent polio virus, and hence protect against this disease.

Other examples of living attenuated vaccines are those of yellow fever and rabies.

Another device is to use for immunisation not the dangerous microbe but a closely related one which is safe yet which gives rise to the production of the same antibodies. The best example of this is **vaccinia** used to vaccinate against smallpox (see pages 72-3).

Unlike non-living vaccines, which have to be injected two or three times to give a lasting immunity, living vaccines need to be administered only once. This is because the living organism remains alive in the tissues for an appreciable time, during which it acts as an effective antigenic stimulus.

Sometimes the use of the words 'vaccinate' and 'inoculate' gives rise to some confusion. They are used interchangeably today.

Artificial Passive Immunisation

So far we have been considering active immunisation, in which the patient is stimulated by the administration of an antigen to produce his own antibodies.

This process takes time. In the case of non-living immunising agents, such as toxoid or bacterial or virus vaccines, at least two injections have to be given, with an interval of a few weeks between them.

Sometimes, however, it is necessary to provide immunity immediately. For example, a child in a family or boarding school may develop diphtheria, and the other children in the group may not have been immunised. They are in serious danger of developing diphtheria within a few days unless they are immunised.

This can be done by giving them injections of antitoxin, that is, of serum containing antibodies made by some other person or animal. Usually, horse antiserum is used for this purpose, though human antiserum may be available in the future. As soon as an adequate amount of antiserum is injected, the child is protected, and the danger averted.

Similarly, patients who have deep and dirty wounds possibly infected with tetanus bacilli may have to be protected against tetanus by anti-tetanic serum (see pages 64-5).

This kind of immunisation is called 'passive', because the patient does not make his own antibody; this antibody is administered 'ready-made' by someone else.

Passive immunisation is only effective for a relatively short period, until the foreign serum containing the antitoxin is eliminated. This may be a few weeks, or only a few days, depending on the individual. If he has had passive immunisation before, he is likely to be 'sensitised' against horse serum, in which case the immunisation will only be likely to last for a few days. This may be all that is required to protect against the danger. For example, the incubation period of diphtheria is only 2-4 days. If the contact has not developed the disease at the end of this time, after the original case of diphtheria has been isolated, he will not develop it. So a few days of protection is enough to meet the immediate danger, though after passive immunisation has worn off the contact will again be susceptible. Active immunisation with toxoid should therefore be started at the same time as or soon after giving the antitoxin, so that permanent protection will result.

Tetanus protection is usually needed for a longer period. The wound harbouring the tetanus bacilli may be of such a kind that it cannot be cleaned out by surgical operation; for instance, a perforating wound of the hand, which surgeons would handle with great care for fear of damaging vital structures. It may remain unhealed for several weeks, with the danger of tetanus developing at any time.

If passive immunisation is relied on in such a case, immunity can only be maintained by repeated doses of antitoxin at approximately weekly intervals.

There is another difficulty about antitoxin treatment. Horse serum, from which most antitoxin is made, is a foreign substance; it contains numerous proteins foreign to the human body against which the patient may react strongly. Illness such as anaphylactic shock or serum sickness, or some other types of allergic reaction, may be the outcome. In some cases, fortunately rare, an immediate and even fatal allergic reaction may occur. So the injection of antitoxin is not without danger. A full dose of antitoxin should never be given without a 'test dose' being given first. The test dose consists of 1/10ml of 1/10 dilution of antitoxin in normal saline, given subcutaneously. After this, the patient should be observed for 20 minutes, to see if any generalised symptoms develop, such as flushing, increase of pulse rate, fall of blood pressure, or a rash.

If such symptoms arise, it is a difficult matter to decide whether or not to proceed with the full dose of antitoxin. This is a medical decision, not one for a nurse.

A syringe containing 1ml of adrenaline, 1/1000, the best method of treating the reactions, should always be at hand when antitoxin is given.

Because of the dangers of tetanus antitoxin prepared from horse serum, many people now consider that it should never be administered, but that one should instead rely on human antitoxin or antibiotics to avert the infection.

Another kind of passive immunisation consists of the administration of human immunoglobulin G (IgG, formerly called gamma glubulin). IgG is the fraction of the serum which contains the antibodies. It comprises about 1/11 of the whole blood. A 'pool' of IgG, prepared from the mixed blood of a number of people, will contain some antibody from all the people in the pool. It will, therefore, give some protection against any of the diseases from which any of these people have suffered in the past. Most human beings have had measles at some time or other, so pooled IgG contains quite an appreciable amount of measles antibody.

IgG is sometimes given to children who have been in contact with measles, to protect them against the disease. This is usually done in the case of very small infants, or weakly children, or children who are ill with some other illness at the time they are in contact with measles. If the IgG is given immediately after the contact, measles will probably be avoided altogether. If it is given at about seven days after contact, it is possible that 'modified' measles will result, consisting of a very mild attack in which the child suffers little more than a rash. Such modified measles is followed by full immunity, whereas complete prevention of the disease is not.

As IgG is made from human serum, not that of horses, it does not give rise to unpleasant reactions as does antitoxin made from horse serum.

IgG specially prepared from actively immunised subjects can be used instead of horse antitoxin for passive protection against tetanus. Anti-vaccinial IgG from recently vaccinated people can also be used to protect smallpox contacts, though it is no substitute for vaccination. However, it is unlikely that there will ever be a sufficient supply of human IgG to meet the need. It is a valuable product and is in short supply. It must not be wasted, but must be used with discretion.

Differences between Active and Passive Immunity

It is useful to summarise the differences between these types of immunisation.

1. Passive immunisation is effective immediately. Active immunisation is effective only after a few days in the case of a living vaccine (e.g. smallpox, BCG), or from the time of the second injection — two or more weeks after the first — in the case of a non-living vaccine.

2. Passive immunisation is short-lasting. Active immunisation is long-lasting, and can be restored to a high level at any time by means of a booster dose.

3. Passive immunisation by horse-antisera carries the risk of allergic reactions. Human IgG is safe in this respect.

For diseases such as diphtheria and tetanus, in which the risk is likely to recur, active immunisation before the likely exposure is obviously the best solution. This means active immunisation in infancy. If a child or adult has to be protected passively because he has not been previously actively immunised, passive immunisation should be followed as soon as possible by active immunisation.

Practical Immunity

In Great Britain, it is recommended that all children should be immunised against:

Diphtheria	**Poliomyelitis**
Tetanus	**Tuberculosis**
Whooping cough	**Measles**

Immunisation against diphtheria, tetanus and whooping cough is best started at any time when the child is between two and six months old. A series of three injections of triple vaccine, at monthly intervals, is the most convenient way of doing this.

Poliomyelitis vaccination may be performed by giving three doses of oral vaccine, at monthly intervals. These may be given at the same time as the triple vaccine, or at a different time; it does not matter.

A booster dose of triple vaccine should be given just before the child is two years old. A further booster dose of diphtheria and tetanus combined toxoid should be given when the child first goes to school.

Revaccination against smallpox should be performed when there is any danger of exposure to smallpox.

BCG vaccination against tuberculosis should be performed at the age of thirteen years or later, provided that the tuberculin reaction is negative.

Immunisation against other diseases:

Influenza: A single dose of killed vaccine gives some protection to about two-thirds of the people vaccinated; this lasts for a few months. Many authorities advocate the vaccination of large groups of people at the beginning of an epidemic.

TAB vaccination against **enteric fever** should be performed when a visit to the Continent of Europe, or any visit to Africa or Asia is contemplated.

Yellow fever and **cholera** immunisation should be given when countries in which these diseases are endemic are to be visited.

Smallpox vaccination used to be recommended for all children. However, this disease has now been eradicated from most countries, so routine vaccination is no longer recommended as it is not completely safe.

Many countries still insist that travellers intending to visit them be vaccinated. It is best to leave an interval of at least four weeks between smallpox vaccination and any other immunisation.

CHAPTER 11

TESTS FOR IMMUNITY

Sometimes it is necessary to know whether people are immune to a particular disease or not. For example, if diphtheria breaks out in a boarding school or children's home, it may be important to know which children are immune and which are susceptible, so that the latter may be protected by immunisation. This can be done by means of the *Schick* test. The test fluid, consisting of diluted diphtheria toxin, is injected into the skin, usually in the forearm. Control fluid, consisting of the toxin heated so as to destroy its toxic effect, is injected into the other arm. Susceptible people have no circulating antitoxin, so the test fluid causes a slight inflammation in the arm in which it has been injected; the control shows nothing. This is a positive reaction. Immune people have circulating antitoxin, which neutralises the toxin, so no reaction is produced in them.

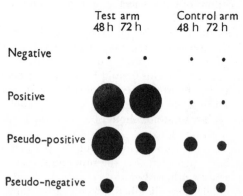

Fig. 35. The Schick test. The reactions are approximately of the size shown

Sometimes people react to materials in the fluid other than the toxin, which is why a control test is used. Such people will get a reaction in the control test as well. Unless there is an appreciable difference between the two sides, the test is negative.

Schick tests are used much less today than in the past, because diphtheria has become very rare, and because most children in this country are known to have been actively immunised.

Delayed Hypersensitivity tests

There is another kind of susceptibility test, much used in looking for immunity to tuberculosis and other diseases. This is the test for allergy or delayed hypersensitivity to the particular microbe. Not only living but killed bacteria can excite the allergic reaction, and so may extracts of the bacteria provided they contain the proteins of the organism. In tuberculin testing, extracts of killed organisms are used, either a crude extract called OT (Old Tuberculin), or a purified protein extract called PPD ('Purified Protein Derivative').

It should be noted that while extracts can be used to produce allergic reactions in people who have already been infected, and can therefore be used for tuberculin testing, extracts and dead bacilli will not make the subjects allergic. Only the living organism will do this. The matter may be put diagrammatically thus:

First contact with living tubercle bacilli ——————▸ Allergy

Thereafter, contact with living bacilli, ——————▸ Allergic
killed bacilli or extract (OT or PPD)   Reaction

It is important to distinguish this test from the tests for direct susceptibility such as the Schick test, as the interpretation of the results is the exact opposite.

The tests for allergy to tuberculosis are called Tuberculin tests. There are many different ways of performing tuberculin tests, which differ only in detail, not in principle. They are mentioned on page 57, and in the table at the end of this chapter.

The principle of the tuberculin tests is as follows. People who become infected with the tubercle bacillus develop an allergy to it, that is to say, their tissues are altered in such a way as to react with a marked local reaction next time they meet the tubercle bacillus. The first time a person is infected with the tubercle bacillus there is hardly any reaction at the site at which the bacillus enters the body, though it may spread through the body and cause chronic or fatal disease. Once this primary infection has occurred, however, the patient becomes **allergic**, that is, his reactions alter. The next time he meets the organism there is a marked local reaction with inflammation and perhaps some tissue necrosis, at the site of entry of the organism. This allergy develops when the primary infection is healed and overcome, or when the patient has been previously infected.

The development of allergy, if the primary infection is overcome, is accompanied by immunity. That is to say, a person who has overcome a primary infection, and become allergic, is immune to another tuberculous infection from outside—though it is possible for an apparently healed infection to flare up again and become reactivated.

Tuberculin tests enable one to separate susceptible people from those who are immune. They are therefore indispensable in deciding which of a group of schoolchildren, medical students, or nurses need to be immunised against tuberculosis and which do not. They are used much more widely than this, in poor countries with a high tuberculosis rate such as India, in

Allergic skin tests similar in principle to the tuberculin test are used in

SOME SKIN TESTS USED IN THE DIAGNOSIS OF INFECTION

Delayed hypersensitivity (allergic) tests — Positive result denotes previous infection

Disease	Test	Method
Tuberculosis	Mantoux	Intradermal injection
	Multiple puncture (Heaf)	Multiple puncture (Heaf gun)
Brucellosis	Brucellin	Intradermal injection
Leprosy	Lepromin	Intradermal injection
Fungous diseases:		
Dermatophytes	Trichophytin	Intradermal injection
Histoplasmosis	Histoplasmin	Intradermal injection
Coccidioidomycosis	Coccidioidin	Intradermal injection
Hydatid disease	Casoni	Intradermal injection
Leishmaniasis	Leishman antigen	Intradermal injection
Virus diseases:		
Lymphogranuloma venereum	Frei	Intradermal injection
Cat-scratch fever	Cat-scratch antigen	Intradermal injection

Direct susceptibility test

Disease	Test	Method
Diphtheria	Schick	Intradermal injection
	Direct susceptibility test to diphtheria toxin. Positive result denotes susceptibility	

enabling doctors to decide which members of the population need to be immunised.

Allergic skin tests, similar in principle to the tuberculin test, are used in the diagnosis of a large number of diseases, such as infections with certain fungi, hydatid cysts, and so on, as shown in the table.

Most people have never been infected with these microbes, but on becoming infected, people become allergic. The allergy tests therefore indicate whether or not infection has occurred. Sometimes they are the only positive finding, and are therefore indispensable in the diagnosis.

Method of performing delayed hypersensitivity tests

A solution containing antigen is injected intradermally (or a Heaf gun or other device is used). The skin is inspected at varying periods after injection for signs of inflammation and induration. 1, 3 or 5 days is the inspection period in most cases.

CHAPTER 12

HYPERSENSITIVITY,
ALLERGY AND AUTO-IMMUNITY

In earlier chapters it was mentioned that when people first become infected with tubercle bacilli, their tissues are altered and will react differently if they meet the bacilli, or extracts of bacilli, for the second time. Any time they meet the tubercle bacilli after the first, their tissues respond after 2-3 days with a marked local reaction with inflammation and sometimes some necrosis.

This kind of reaction is called a delayed hypersensitivity reaction, and is due to the action of cells called T-lymphocytes which are produced by the thymus (T) gland. It illustrates an important point, namely, that when human beings first meet a bacterium, or indeed any antigen, and start to develop antibodies to it, they are never quite the same again. Their tissues become permanently altered, or sensitised, and the next time they meet the bacterium, or antigen, they react in a different manner from the first.

Sometimes this altered or allergic reaction may be of value to the patient in helping him to resist disease. Thus, allergy in tuberculosis brings immunity with it. Moreover, the detection of allergic reactions can be used as a means of detecting previous infection against a number of microbes, as listed on the Table in Chapter 11 (page 140).

The allergic reaction in tuberculosis is complicated and has a number of components. One of them is an increase in the blood supply to old tuberculous lesions. This may cause the spread into the blood-stream of tubercle bacilli which had, until then, been securely encapsulated within the lesion. In this way, an old infection may be 'lit-up' and this may result in a spread of the disease. This is particularly likely to happen in the lung, where a secondary infection with tubercle bacilli in the lung may lead to the development of further inflammatory or necrotic nodules.

Sometimes, therefore, allergic reactions are not at all beneficial, but may be positively harmful.

Anaphylaxis. The development of the tuberculin type of reaction is fairly constant in different individuals; people do not differ very much. Individuals do vary greatly, however, in the way in which they become sensitised to other antigens. Sometimes contact with an antigen to which the person is sensitised may cause an immediate acute hypersensitivity reaction. This is because the serum contains larger amounts than normal of a globulin called **IgE**. The reaction takes the form of a rapid fall in blood pressure, a rapid pulse, a feeling of collapse, with possibly the appearance of wheals or papules on the skin, and an attack of asthma. This is **anaphylactic shock**. Such reactions may be extremely serious, and indeed can be rapidly fatal.

Anaphylactic shock sometimes occurs when people are given injections of antitoxin made from horse serum such as anti-tetanus and anti-diphtheria toxin. The way to avoid them is by giving a 'test dose' of diluted antigen subcutaneously and watching the patient for half an hour, before proceeding to the main dose. Both the test dose and the main dose must be given under medical supervision.

However, even it a test dose is given an anaphylactic reaction may occur. This is an acute medical emergency, and should be treated by a doctor. There should always be a bottle of 1/1000 adrenalin solution, and a syringe and needles, ready for such an emergency. Adrenalin counteracts the action of histamine, which is the poisonous substance liberated by the sensitised tissues and causing anaphylactic shock.

Anaphylactic reactions sometimes occur after injections of penicillin or other drugs. People who are known to be allergic to penicillin cannot have penicillin injections, but must be treated by some other antibiotic.

Atopic reactions. It is well known that some people are 'sensitive', or rather, hypersensitive, to certain foods such as shellfish or strawberries, and become ill if they eat these; they may come out in a rash. The same thing applies to cosmetics, shampoo materials, disinfectants and so on; some people are 'hypersensitive' and develop allergic reactions when they come into contact with these substances. They do this because they develop antibodies against them. 'Hay fever' is a similar reaction; people who suffer from it are hypersensitive to pollen and contact with this produces an acute catarrh of the respiratory tract.

These reactions are called by various names, such as 'atopic reactions', and 'idiosyncrasies'; they are usually trivial. They can easily be avoided once the reaction is known about, for it is usually specific, that is to say, it is only particular chemical substances that excite it.

People may develop these atopic reactions at any time. They may develop them against drugs such as penicillin or against substances which they use in their daily work, such as paint or chemicals. The results of this kind of sensitisation may obviously be very unfortunate and inconvenient and may even make it necessary for a person to change his occupation.

Hypersensitivity Diseases. Another variety of the same abnormality is found when people are sensitive to a wide range of substances. Exposure to one of these may result in a definite illness — a chest illness, asthma; a skin reaction, urticaria; and so on. Asthma is a common disease; it is usually due to sensitisation, that is to say the development of abnormal antibodies, to a particular substance or group of substances. Asthmatic attacks vary greatly in severity; they may be trivial, but they can be extremely serious and disabling, and may even continue until the patient dies in an attack ('status asthmaticus').

Infantile eczema is another example of the same type of illness, though in this case the cause is usually not known. The infant's skin is extremely sensitive, and becomes inflamed easily after contact with a variety of substances. It may become secondarily infected, and the child may be very ill as a result. Children mostly grow out of this complaint, but they may do so only to develop an allergic disease in some other part of the body, for example, asthma.

The skin may remain abnormally sensitive throughout the patient's life. If this happens, any injection in the skin may result in a widespread illness. Eczematous subjects have to be particularly careful about smallpox vaccination, and vaccination should be avoided, if possible, while the patient is suffering from any active eczematous lesion.

It is possible, in some of these cases of asthma or eczema, to **desensitise** the patient by removing some or all of the abnormal antibody that is the cause of the trouble. This can only be done if the antigen is known, and to find this out, skin tests against extracts of particular substances can be performed. If, for example, the patient is allergic to feathers, an injection into the skin of an extract of feathers will produce a local inflammatory reaction. It may then be possible to desensitise the patient by repeated minute small doses of feather extract, too small to produce an allergic reaction, but big enough to neutralise some of the antibody and bring about its removal.

This allergic tendency often runs in families and is hereditary. It seems to represent a general tendency on the part of an individual. Thus, people who are eczematous may also get occasional attacks of asthma, and vice versa. Emotional disturbances may also play a part in starting attacks.

Another example of the same type of reaction is that which people may develop after injections of antiserum for passive immunisation against diphtheria, or tetanus, or any other illness in which antiserum is used. This is usually an allergic reaction to the horse protein in the antiserum. It may take the form of an immediate anaphylactic reaction as mentioned above.

The reaction may, on the other hand, be delayed for several days, after which the patient may develop 'serum sickness'. This is an illness in which there are a rise in temperature, pains in the joints, headache, and often an eruption at the site of the original injection. It subsides on its own after a few days, and is rarely serious.

An important rule is — **always take notice if a patient tells you that he is allergic or abnormally sensitive to any particular substance**. Never, in any circumstances, ignore any warning a patient may give you; usually he knows only too well the consequences of contact with any particular substance, and these may be serious, or even fatal.

There is an entirely different kind of allergic disease in which the patient develops an abnormally large amount of antibody against a particular micro-organism, namely *Streptococcus pyogenes*, the cause of acute tonsillitis (see page 41). Some weeks after streptococcal infection, the patient may become seriously ill with either rheumatic fever or acute nephritis, diseases caused by damage in the cells of either the heart, joints, or kidneys due to the abnormal antibody.

The effects of rheumatic fever often last, in one form or another, throughout the patient's life; serious heart disease may result. Nephritis is less often lasting in its effects; none the less, it is a serious illness.

It is now known that almost any type of rheumatic illness, for example, rheumatoid arthritis, may be due to a similar mechanism, the development of abnormal antibodies against Streptococcus pyogenes.

Rheumatic fever usually occurs in children, and it is important so far as possible to prevent children from getting attacks of streptococcal infection; this is the main reason why tonsils are removed so often in childhood. Children who have had an attack of rheumatic fever or acute nephritis must be guarded against further attacks. This may be done by giving them small doses of an antibiotic by mouth every day, for example a single 250mg tablet of phenethicillin (Broxil). This is sufficient to prevent the streptococci ever getting a foothold and causing disease.

In recent years it has become known that many other diseases whose origin was previously unknown are due to the development of abnormal antibody. Examples are disseminated lupus erythematosus and periarteritis nodosa. Also the development of **auto-immune** disease has a similar background. In auto-immune disease, the patient develops antibodies against a natural product of his own body. The best known of these diseases is **Hashimoto's disease**, a form of thyroid inflammation, in which the patient develops antibodies against thyroid secretion. The result is that the thyroid gland becomes inflamed, and the body becomes deficient in thyroid secretion which is neutralised by the antibody. It is probable that some diseases of other organs are also due to the development of auto-antibodies. It may seem a far cry from sensitivity to shellfish or mascara to rheumatic fever and Hashimoto's disease. But in fact all the conditions mentioned in this chapter have one basic thing in common, the abnormal development of antibodies, which cause the patient harm.

CHAPTER 13

THE USE OF
SEROLOGICAL TESTS IN DIAGNOSIS

Serological tests are much used in the pathology laboratory in the diagnosis of infective disease. They may be used in one of two ways.

The first way is to help in the identification of a microbe. For example, the best method of distinguishing between the large number of different bacilli of the salmonella group is by serological tests. The reactions of the bacilli are tested against specific antisera obtained by immunising rabbits with each particular organism separately. The microbes are **agglutinated** (clumped) by the specific antiserum but not by any other antiserum.

Thus when a patient is suspected of having typhoid or some other variety of enteric fever, and a suspicious bacterium is isolated from his stool, it is identified by testing with specific antisera in this way, to see which one agglutinates it. If it is agglutinated by the typhoid but not by the paratyphoid antisera, it is a typhoid bacillus, not a paratyphoid, and so on.

In a similar manner, viruses may be tested against specific antisera by a number of different methods. One method is the **precipitin test**. Some virus antigens are soluble, and form a precipitate with specific antisera if they are allowed to react with them. Fluid from pocks in suspected smallpox may be tested against smallpox antiserum to see if it gives a precipitate; if it does, the virus present in the pocks and causing the infection is smallpox virus. Alternatively, the virus may be tested by various sera to see which of them neutralises its effect on susceptible tissue cells. This is the **neutralisation test.**

The other way in which serological tests may be used in the diagnosis of disease is by examining patients' sera to see if they have developed antibodies against particular microbes. For example, in a suspected case of typhoid or paratyphoid it sometimes happens that attempts to isolate the microbe from the patient's stool or blood are unsuccessful. However, if the patient has developed, in his serum, antibodies against the typhoid bacillus, and these have increased in quantity greatly during the course of his illness, it is usually a fair assumption that the infection from which the patient is suffering is typhoid. In the case of typhoid and related infections, antibodies can be detected quite easily because they agglutinate or clump the bacteria, an effect which is clearly visible. The test is performed by taking the patient's serum, and making 'serial dilutions' of it, such as 1/20; 1/40, and so on, in small tubes. To each of these tubes, a suspension of killed typhoid bacilli is added. If antibody is present in the serum, the bacilli will be agglutinated or clumped. By this means not only can the presence of antibody be demonstrated, but also an indication of their concentration, by observing how much the patient's serum has to be diluted before the clumping is no longer visible. The highest dilution at which agglutination is observed gives the 'titre' of the serum. This test is sometimes called the Widal reaction.

Patients often enter hospital suffering from unexplained pyrexia. A Widal reaction, in which the serum is tested for antibodies not only against typhoid but against other possible infections also, such as paratyphoid, *Salmonella typhi-murium*, and the brucellas, may give the only positive information about the nature of the infection.

A more intricate type of test, which is of much wider application than the agglutination or Widal test, is the **Complement Fixation Test** (CFT). This is technically rather complicated though, like all serological tests, it depends on the detection of specific antibodies in the patient's serum by letting this react with an antigen. The **Wassermann** test for syphilis is a complement fixation test, and similar tests are also used for the diagnosis of gonorrhoea, and a wide variety of other infections including many virus infections. In fact, the complement fixation reaction can be adapted to the diagnosis of any type of infective disease in which the causative organism has been isolated. It, too, can be performed as a quantitative test by observing the highest dilution of serum to give a positive reaction. Other serological tests are devised to suit particular forms of infection. Thus, one of the properties of haemolytic streptococci is that they lyse, or destroy, red blood cells. This they do by virtue of a toxin called the **haemolysin**. Patients infected with these organisms develop an antibody to the haemolysin called the **anti-streptolysin**. A serological test much used in the diagnosis of suspected streptococcal infection is the titration of anti-streptolysin.

This test is also of value in the diagnosis of rheumatic conditions, which are known to be due to allergy to haemolytic streptococci. If a patient with a subacute or chronic rheumatoid condition persistently has a high anti-streptolysin (**ASO**) titre, this strongly suggests streptococcal allergy.

Another special test used in suspected rheumatic conditions and in other inflammatory states is the **Rheumatoid (RA) factor test.** This is also known by other names which are given in the table at the end of this chapter.

Precipitin tests, in which soluble antigens extracted from microbes are allowed to react with a patient's serum, are also much used. If the serum contains specific antibodies, a precipitate will form. The **Kahn** test, which is often used together with the Wasserman test in the diagnosis of syphilis, is a precipitin test.

Precipitin tests are often carried out in a medium of agar gel, which slows the reaction down and makes it easier to detect. The antigen and the suspected antibody are allowed to flow together through the agar from opposite directions. When they meet and react, a precipitate occurs which appears as opaque lines in the agar. This is the **agar-gel diffusion** technique.

Agar-gel diffusion techniques are also used in the diagnosis of auto-immune diseases. Another technique which has been developed in recent years is **immuno-electrophoresis**. This depends on the fact that

SOME EXAMPLES OF SEROLOGICAL TESTS USED
IN THE DIAGNOSIS OF DISEASE

To detect microbes in pathological specimens

Method	Examples
Agglutination	Typhoid, paratyphoid and other salmonellas, dysentery bacilli, whooping cough, B. coli, Streptococci
Haemagglutination	Hepatitis B
Precipitin	Viruses e.g. smallpox
Neutralisation	Viruses e.g. smallpox

To detect or measure antibodies in serum

Method	Examples
Agglutination	Widal test in suspected typhoid and paratyphoid, also brucellosis, typhus, leptospirosis and 'cold agglutination' in suspected virus pneumonia
Complement fixation	Wassermann test for syphilis, also in many other infections such as gonorrhoea and various bacterial and virus diseases. A number of specialised tests for syphilis have been developed in recent years
Anti-streptolysin	Streptococci
Anti-staphylolysin	Staphylococci
Treponema immobilisation test	In suspected syphilis
Haemagglutination-inhibition test	In influenza
Fluorescent antibody tests	In various diseases
Radio-immune	Australia antigen

Empirical tests whose mechanism is not fully understood

Paul-Bunnell reaction	In suspected glandular fever (infectious mononucleosis)
Rheumatoid factor (RA) test, also called Rose-Waaler or Differential sheep cell agglutination test (DAT)	For rheumatoid arthritis factor
Antinuclear factor test } LE cell test }	In suspected systemic lupus erythematosis

different protein fractions of serum diffuse along a suitable medium at different speeds when an electric current is passed through them. However, a further discussion of this rather specialised topic is beyond the scope of this book.

Precipitin tests are widely used for medico-legal purposes. For example, the specific antigens of the red blood cells are soluble and give rise to precipitin formation. Precipitin tests may be used to test blood stains to see which species of animal they come from, or, if human, to which blood group they belong. They may thus help to identify murderers or their victims.

There are various difficulties about the interpretation of all these tests so far as the diagnosis of a particular illness is concerned. The first is that antibodies may be present in the patient's serum as a result of a past illness, or as a result of past sub-clinical infection, and may not have anything to do with the present illness at all. This difficulty can be overcome to some extent by taking 'paired sera' from the patient — one sample as early as possible in the illness, and a second sample at least a fortnight later. If a marked rise in antibodies to one particular microbe occurs in that fortnight, that is probably the microbe causing the infection. If there is no appreciable change of antibody levels during the fortnight, the antibodies present are probably left over from some previous infection.

Antibody tests on the patient's serum are valuable not only in the diagnosis of illness, but also in assessing the results of immunisation. For example, about the only possible way of seeing whether a particular polio vaccine is likely to be effective or not (apart from seeing whether immunised patients actually get the illness) is by estimating the antibody in the serum after immunisation.

CHAPTER 14

ANTIBIOTICS IN THE
TREATMENT OF INFECTION

Introduction

The fact that it is necessary to include this chapter in a book about
bacteriology in an indication of the great progress that has been made in
the past 40 years. Before World War II the treatment of most infections
was symptomatic and empirical. There was no specific treatment, and all
that the doctor could do was to help the natural defences of the body by
keeping the patient warm, at rest, suitably stimulated, and so on.

It is difficult today to realise just how serious in those days were the
consequences of quite trivial injuries. A surgeon who pricked his finger
during a minor operation for opening an abscess could do nothing effective
to stop the course of the infection which followed. Once the injury took
place, the disease started on its course, which might well be fatal. Lobar
pneumonia was a dreaded disease in which, after some days of mounting
illness, the patient passed into a state of 'crisis' which ended either in
recovery or death. During the recovery stage, empyema might occur,
adding weeks or months of serious and painful illness. Pneumococcal
meningitis and tuberculosis meningitis were almost invariably fatal;
recovery from these diseases hardly ever occurred. Typhoid fever was often
fatal and nothing effective could be done to help the patient. A diagnosis
of tuberculosis always meant months of serious disabling illness in a special
hospital or sanatorium, away from family and friends, and the prospect of
being an invalid for life. Ordinary household and gardening accidents
were often fraught with the most terrible consequences of septicaemia,
cellulitis, multiple abscess formation, deformity and death.

These serious consequences can still follow infections, but this seldom
happens. The change is entirely due to the development of antibiotic and
chemotherapeutic drugs.

In 1928 Alexander Fleming noticed that a fungus spore chanced to
contaminate one of the culture plates in his laboratory at St Mary's
Hospital, and prevented the growth of staphylococci which he was
culturing. This observation, followed up and investigated, led eventually
to the discovery of penicillin, the first and most important of all the
antibiotic drugs.

Before the full development of penicillin, in the 1940s, sulphonamide
drugs had been developed and brought into wide use in the years 1938 and
1939. These were a tremendous breakthrough, and 'M & B 693', the trade
name of sulphapyridine, a sulphonamide drug, became a household word
in the treatment of pneumococcal and other infections which suddenly
ceased to be a serious menace to life. Domagk, the German scientist, was

149

chiefly responsible for the early development of the sulphonamides. A second important breakthrough was the development of penicillin by Florey and Chain in Oxford in 1939 and later years. A third was the development of streptomycin by Waksman, in 1944, which made possible the drug treatment of tuberculosis.

After this, a systematic study by big industrial research establishments led to the introduction of the tetracyclines, erythromycin, and the other antibiotics used today. Another important advance was the discovery of the method of breaking up the molecule of penicillin, which has led in recent years to the introduction of even more powerful antibiotics.

The discovery of drugs effective against pathogenic fungi, namely, nystatin, amphotericin B, griseofulvin, and others, has also occurred in recent years. There remains the conquest of virus disease, and it is possible that the discovery of interferon, a substance produced by virus which prevents the growth of other viruses, may turn out to have been a decisive breakthrough here.

The drama of the discovery of the drugs named above is still fresh in the minds of most middle-aged people. However, the use of chemical substances to treat infection systematically started much earlier. Paul Ehrlich first used arsenical drugs successfully for the treatment of syphilis and other spirochaetal infections in the early part of this century. He coined the term **chemotherapy** to denote this type of treatment. Antibiotics are chemotherapeutic agents which are derived from living organisms such as moulds. Nowadays, the terms antibiotic therapy and chemotherapy are used almost interchangeably. For the sake of convenience, in this chapter, the entire range of chemotherapeutic and antibiotic drugs are referred to as antibiotics.

Review of Antibiotics

At present a large number of antibiotics are available, and the number is constantly increasing. Those in use at the time of writing are considered below briefly under the following headings:

> Sulphonamides
> Penicillins and synthetic penicillins
> Cephalosporin
> Streptomycin and its derivatives
> Tetracyclines
> Chloramphenicol
> Erythromycin
> Fucidin
> Other antibacterial antibiotics
> Antifungal antibiotics

Sulphonamides

These were the first modern successful chemotherapeutic drugs, and are usually taken by mouth. They have been much refined since the early days of 'M & B 693' (sulphapyridine), a most effective drug which however had many undesirable side effects.

Today numerous sulphonamides are available for treating a wide variety of infections. On the whole, they have been overshadowed by antibiotics, which is a pity as the modern sulphonamides are effective and relatively harmless drugs. They are recommended for the following:

Meningococcal infections.
Urinary infections with *E. coli* and other coliforms.
Pneumococcal infections ⎫   Sulphonamides are as effective as any
Streptococcal infections ⎭   other drugs.
Gonorrhoea. Sulphonamides may be effective.

Bacillary dysentery. 'Insoluble' sulphonamides, given in large doses, are best for this disease; the large dose and their insolubility enable high concentrations to be attained in the intestine.

Sulphonamides recommended for general use: (the dose stated is the average adult dose).
Sulphadimidine (Sulphamezathine).
    Dose: 3g followed by 1-1.5g every six hours. For urinary infections, 2g followed by 0.5-1g every 6-8 hours.
Sulphadiazine.
    Dose: As for Sulphadimidine.

Sulphonamides recommended for urinary infections
Sulphafurazole (Sulphisoxalose, Gantrisin).
    Dose: 3g followed by 1.5g every six hours.
Sulphasomidine (Elkosin).
    Dose: 3g followed by 1.5g every six hours.
Sulphamethizole (Urolucosil).
    Dose: 0.25-0.5g every 4-6 hours.

Sulphonamides of low solubility for treatment of bacillary dysentery
Succinylsulphathiazole (sulphasuxidine).
    Dose: 5-10g daily.
Phthalylsulphathiazole (sulphathalidine).
    Dose: 10-20g daily.
These can be given in large doses as shown.

Long-acting sulphonamides
Sulphamethoxypyridazine ⎫
  (Midicel)   ⎪ These are quickly absorbed and
Sulphadimethoxine   ⎬ slowly excreted.
  (Madribon)   ⎪
Sulphaphenazole (Orisulf) ⎭
    Dose: Only one dose need by given daily. 1g on the first day followed by 0.5g on subsequent days.

Sulphonamide mixtures are also sometimes used—sulphatriad and trisulphonamide.

Trimethoprim is often given in combination with a sulphonamide to enhance the effect.

Penicillins

Today there are many derivatives of the original penicillin which was discovered by Fleming and developed by Florey and Chain. The original penicillin is: **benzyl penicillin** (Penicillin G), a soluble drug which diffuses readily into tissues. It is only active when given by injection, not when taken by mouth. To maintain an efective blood concentration, it is necessary to do one of the following:

1. Give injections every eight hours.
2. Give a drug such as Probenecid which interferes with the excretion of penicillin by the kidneys.
3. Give penicillin compounded with a substance which delays its absorption, such as procaine penicillin, benethamine and benzathine penicillin.

Phenoxymethyl penicillin (Penicillin V). This is a derivative of penicillin which is stable in acid and can therefore be given by mouth.

The following bacteria are sensitive to Penicillins G and V:

Staphylococci (but about 70% in hospitals are resistant)	Meningococci
	Clostridia
Streptococci	Diphtheria bacilli
Pneumococci	Anthrax bacilli
Gonococci	Spirochaetes

Other bacteria may also be sensitive.

Disadvantages

1. **Allergy.** Many people who have been sensitised by previous contact with penicillin are allergic. When penicillin is administered they may have one of two types of reaction, either an immediate profound state of anaphylactic shock, or a delayed reaction of the serum sickness type (see page 143). Asthmatics, or patients with a history of any other type of allergic disease, are a special risk.

Nurses and others who handle penicillin are liable to develop allergy to it. They should avoid direct contact with powders, solutions, and sprays containing penicillin.

Before any patient is given an injection of penicillin, he should be asked about sensitivity. **On no account should penicillin be administered to a patient with a history of sensitivity.** The result may be fatal.

Dose: This depends on the nature and site of infection. The minimum likely to be useful are approximately:

300 000 units four-hourly of Penicillin G by injection.

300 000 units twelve-hourly of Penicillin V.

0.25g four-hourly (by mouth) of Penicillin V.

Much larger doses are frequently given.

The Intrathecal dosage is usually 10 000 units.

2. **Superinfection.** Another danger is that the patient may contract a second infection or superinfection with a microbe resistant to penicillin, such as resistant staphylococci. These are resistant because they produce an enzyme, penicillinase, which destroys penicillin. Other possible causes of superinfection are pathogenic fungi such as *Candida albicans.*

Synthetic Penicillins

A great advance in chemistry made possible the discovery and isolation a few years ago of the penicillin nucleus, 6-amino-penicillanic acid. This enabled many new penicillin compounds to be manufactured, with properties not possessed by the early derivatives of Penicillin G. These are called the synthetic penicillins.

The synthetic penicillins useful in medicine are those which possess one or more of the following properties:

1. Resistance to acid, so that drugs are effective when taken by mouth.

   e.g. Phenethicillin (Broxil)   Ampicillin (Penbritin)

       Propicillin (Brocillin)   Cloxacillin (Orbenin)

       Phenbenicillin (Penspek)   Amoxycillin

2. Resistance to penicillinase, so that the drug is effective against penicillin-resistant staphylococci.

   e.g. Methicillin (Celbenin) Cloxacillin (Orbenin) Flucloxacillin

3. Activity against gram-negative bacteria, so that the drug can be used in the treatment of typhoid, other salmonella infections, haemophilus infections, and the like.

   e.g. Ampicillin (Penbritin). (See Table on pages 157-8).

       Carbenicillin — particularly active against *Ps. aeruginosa* and Proteus.

There is thus a rich variety of penicillins to choose from today.

The usual dose of these drugs is 250-500mg every four or six hours, by mouth or by injection.

Cephalosporins. This is a group of antibiotics useful in the treatment of:

1. Patients who are allergic to penicillin but would otherwise be treated with penicillin.

2. Penicillin-resistant staphylococcal infections.

Examples are **Cephaloridine, Cephalothin**, and **Cephalexin.**

Streptomycin

Streptomycin is active against tubercle bacilli. However, these readily become resistant to it, so in the treatment of tuberculosis streptomycin is usually used in combination with one or two other drugs such as **Para-aminosalicylic acid (PAS), Isoniazid (INAH), Rifampicin,** and **Ethambutol.** Anti-tuberculous treatment may have to continue for many months.

Streptomycin is not absorbed from the gut and must be given by injection. The usual dose is ½ or 1g per day.

Streptomycin is relatively toxic. It affects the middle and inner ears if taken too long or in excessive dosage. The result is disturbance of equilibrium or deafness, which may be permanent. The danger of these complications arising must always be borne in mind when patients are treated with streptomycin.

In addition to its activity against tubercle bacilli, streptomycin is also active against many gram-negative and some gram-positive organisms. However, owing to its toxicity, it is rarely used for these purposes.

CLINICALLY USEFUL PENICILLINS

Name	Trade names	Important properties
Benzyl penicillin	Crystapen Eskacillin Falapen Solupen	Given by injection
Phenoxymethyl penicillin	Calcipen V Compocillin VK Crystapen V Dystaquaine V-K Econopen V Icipen V Penavlon V Pencicals Penicillin V Stabillin V-K V-cil-K	Can be taken by mouth
Phenethicillin	Broxil	Can be taken by mouth
Propicillin	Brocillin Ultrapen	Can be taken by mouth
Phenbenicillin	Penspek	Can be taken by mouth
Ampicillin Amoxycillin (Amoxil)	Penbritin	Active against many Gram-negative bacilli Can be taken by mouth
Carbenicillin	Pyopen	Active in most Pseudomonas and Proteus infections
Methicillin	Celbenin Staphcillin	Penicillinase-resistant Given by injection
Cloxacillin Flucloxacillin (Floxapen)	Orbenin	Penicillinase-resistant Can be taken by mouth

Dihydrostreptomycin is a less toxic derivative of streptomycin.

Gentamicin is particularly useful in urinary infections due to *Ps. aeruginosa.*

Neomycin, Framycetin, Kanamycin, Paromomycin and **Tobramycin** are derived from related species of streptomyces.

Tetracyclines

The tetracyclines are drugs active against a wide range of microbes including some of the larger visuses. For this reason they are called 'broad-spectrum antibiotics'. They can all be taken by mouth, and there is little difference in their antibacterial ranges. The most important are:

> Tetracycline
> Chlortetracycline (Aureomycin)
> Oxytetracycline (Terramycin)
> Dimethylchlortetracycline

Dose. 0.25mg four-hourly by mouth.

Range of activity. Most types of bacterial infection, also active against rickettsias and Chlamydia. No effect against fungi.

Side effects. These are not common, but may be troublesome. Nausea, vomiting and diarrhoea occur from irritation of the mucous membrane of the gut.

Treatment with the tetracyclines also always carries the risk of 'super-infections' with microbes resistant to these drugs, even though the original infection, for which treatment has been given, may be satisfactorily dealt with. Many strains of staphylococci are resistant, especially in hospitals. Staphylococcal pneumonia and staphylococcal enterocolitis are hazards of tetracycline therapy.

Another possible danger is infection with fungi, of which *Candida albicans*, the thrush fungus, is the commonest.

Chloramphenicol (Chloromycetin)

This is a broad-spectrum antibiotic. It was the first drug to show any appreciable activity against the rickettsias of typhus and it is also most useful in the treatment of typhoid. Unfortunately its use can be dangerous (see below) and it is not much used now. As the range of activity of the tetracyclines is similar to that of chloramphenicol, the former are used in preference to it whenever possible.

Dose. 250mg four-hourly by mouth.

Side effects. When taken for long periods, that is to say several weeks, chloramphenicol may cause severe depression of the bone marrow, leading to agranulocytosis or even aplastic anaemia.

Erythromycin can be taken by mouth and is active against gram-positive cocci. It can often be used to treat infections by staphylococci which are penicillin-resistant. However, staphylococci soon acquire resistance to it. It is also useful in the treatment of streptococcal or pneumococcal infections when the patient is allergic to penicillin.

Fucidin is often effective in staphylococcal infections resistant to penicillin.

Two other very useful drugs in the treatment of *E. coli* urinary infections are **Nalidixic acid** and **Nitrofurantoin.**

There is a very large number of other antibacterial antibiotics, and the number is constantly increasing. It is impossible even to mention them all in a brief review, though many are listed on the Table below. Most bacterial infections may now be successfully treated by antibiotics. There are, however, still some difficult infections to treat, especially those by resistant staphylococci, by Pseudomonas, and by Proteus.

Antifungal Antibiotics

Griseofulvin is active against dermatophyte infections, and is particularly useful in those which cannot be treated easily by local application of ointments, etc., such as infections of the finger nails and toenails. It is taken by mouth. Treatment must be continued for a long period — several weeks or even months.

Nystatin. This substance is active against *Candida albicans* infections. It can be taken by mouth in the form of tablets or lozenges for the treatment of oral or intestinal thrush. Nystatin pessaries are probably the best method of treating vaginal thrush.

Amphotericin B is active against many types of fungus infection. However, it is toxic when given by injection and should be used with care; there is danger of permanent kidney damage. Amphotericin B can also be used in local applications for the treatment of candida infections.

5-Fluorocytosine. Active in many types of fungus infection and less toxic than Amphotericin B.

Clotrimazole. Active in many types of fungus infection.

CHOICE OF ANTIBIOTICS IN THE TREATMENT OF INFECTIONS

The organism isolated should always be tested for sensitivity

Infection	1st choice	2nd and 3rd choice	Remarks
Staphylococci	Pencillin (if sensitive) Flucloxacillin (if patient is sensitive to pencillins: Fucidin + lincomycin) Fucidin (if penicillin resistant)	Tetracyclines Erythromycin Fucidin	
Streptococci Pneumococci Gonococci Meningococci	Penicillin	Tetracyclines Sulphonamides Erythromycin	
Haemophilus	Ampicillin	Tetracyclines	
Whooping cough	Tetracyclines	Chloramphenicol	
Diphtheria	Pencillin		+ Antitoxin
E. coli Klebsiella	Ampicillin Tetracyclines Sulphonamides or other antibiotics according to sensitivity tests may be given alone or in combination with Trimethoprim Nalidixic acid Nitrofurantoin		
Dysentery — bacillary	Sulphonamides	Ampicillin Tetracyclines	
Dysentery — amoebic	Metronidazole	Emetine compounds	
Typhoid and Paratyphoid	Chloramphenicol	Ampicillin Tetracyclines	
Brucella	Tetracyclines with Sulphonamides or Streptomycin		
Tuberculosis	Streptomycin Isoniazid PAS combined		A combination of drugs should always be used
Anthrax	Penicillin	Tetracyclines	
Clostridial infections	Penicillin	Tetracyclines	+ Antitoxin + Surgery

Infection	1st choice	2nd and 3rd choice	Remarks
Proteus	{ Kanamycin Carbenicillin Co-trimoxazole Streptomycin Micin		
Pseudomonas	{ Neomycin Polymyxins Gentamicin Carbenicillin		
Syphilis	Penicillin		
Leptospira	Penicillin	{ Tetracyclines Erythromycin	
Other spirochaetes	Penicillin	Tetracyclines	
Yersinia pestis	Streptomycin	{ Sulphonamides Chloramphenicol	Combinations may be useful
Rickettsias	Tetracyclines	Chloramphenicol	
Psittacosis	Tetracyclines		
Smallpox (prevention)	Thiosemicarbazones		Vaccination the most important measure
Other viruses	None		
Dermatophytes:	Local: various applications Systemic: Griseofulvin		
Candida infections	Local: Nystatin or 5-fluorocytosine or Amphotericin B Systemic: Amphotericin B		Amphotericin B injections may be toxic
Other systemic fungal infections	5-fluorocytosine or Amphotericin B		Amphotericin B injections may be toxic

CHAPTER 15

THE COLLECTION OF SPECIMENS FOR BACTERIOLOGICAL EXAMINATION

Bacteriological diagnosis is made by **cultural examination** — identifying microbes grown from specimens taken from the patient — and by **serological examination** — looking for antibodies to various microbes in the patient's serum.

Cultural Examination

The following are the specimens most often used:

Swabs — of cotton wool, on a wooden or plastic stick. These must of course be sterile. They are used for surface specimens such as the skin, mouth, conjunctiva, and vagina, infected wounds, and pus from boils and abscesses.

Urine — usually 'clean' or 'midstream' specimens. The same specimen may be used for microscopical and chemical examination.

Dip slides and similar methods are useful for rapid sampling.

Sputum, faeces, and **body fluids** from internal organs, for example **cerebrospinal fluid ('CSF')** in suspected cases of meningitis, **pleural fluid** in cases of pleurisy or empyema, and **peritoneal fluid** in some cases of peritonitis. These internal specimens are taken by a doctor, usually under local anaesthesia.

Important Points about Collecting Specimens

1. The specimen must be taken in a sterile manner to avoid contamination.

2. The swab, collecting bottle, or container must be sterile.

3. Be careful to take the correct type of specimen. It is no use taking a sample of saliva if sputum is required. When taking swabs, make sure that the diseased area is swabbed and not the surrounding area, which may be infected with normal commensal organisms but not those causing the disease.

4. Take care not to contaminate the specimen. It should be exposed for the least possible time before being placed in the collecting bottle or tube. This should be properly closed with a sterile cotton-wool plug or screw cap, so that the specimen can be transported to the laboratory without fear of contamination.

5. Taking the specimen must not harm the patient. This is why catheter specimens of urine are not often taken, as they occasionally cause infection.

6. **Make sure the specimen is correctly labelled with the patient's full name.** Many serious mistakes have been caused through not doing this **as soon as possible** after taking the specimen.

7. Specimens must be taken to the laboratory for examination as soon as possible. Some microbes are delicate and die rapidly if the specimen is left to stand at room temperature or refrigerated. If it is impossible for the specimen to be delivered to the laboratory immediately, because it is taken at night or during the week-end, it should be kept safe in a suitable place at the correct temperature. Some laboratories issue special 'transport media' or 'conservation media' into which the specimen should be taken. Instructions about how to deal with the various types of specimen should be obtained from the laboratory and kept in the ward office where they can easily be consulted.

Each specimen should be sent to the laboratory with a fully completed request form signed by a doctor.

8. When an urgent result is required, or in the case of CSF and other body fluids which are particularly valuable specimens, it is important to make sure that the laboratory receives them at a time when they can be examined satisfactorily.

For most laboratories, the last hour of the working day should be avoided; it is a 'rush-hour'. **Specimens should be sent to the laboratory as early in the day as possible**; and a phone call to warn the laboratory to expect a particularly important specimen will often help. Few laboratories are able to provide a 24-hour service, and specimens are often wasted because they arrive at the laboratory too late or after the staff have gone home.

9. Some specimens are dangerous to handle. Plastic bags, which can be sealed, should be used to transport these.

10. When a specimen is discarded, it should be disposed of safely and hygienically.

Notes on some specimens

Pus: Send a few drops of the actual pus whenever possible. If a swab is used, make sure that this is taken from the pus and not the surrounding skin.

Throat Swabs: Be sure that you actually wipe the surface of the tonsil or the back of the throat; this must be done quickly, yet gently, so as to avoid making the patient 'gag'. Avoid touching the tongue or the inside of the mouth to prevent contamination by 'commensal' organisms.

Nasal Swabs: Take the specimen quickly to avoid disturbing the patient more than is absolutely necessary.

Post-Nasal Swabs: Often used in suspected whooping cough. The swab, which is bent at the end (see Fig. 23, page 53) is passed behind the uvula to the post-nasal mucous membrane. This has to be done quickly and gently.

Vaginal, urethral, and wound swabs: Unless they are taken straight to the laboratory immediately, these should be broken into transport medium.

Sputum: The specimen should include lumps of mucoid sputum and not merely watery saliva. It is best collected in a wide-mouthed disposable container with a screw cap, so that the specimen will not spill when being taken to the laboratory.

Urine: Urine passed in the usual way is always contaminated by microbes present on the skin surrounding the urinary meatus. For cultural examination, a clean or midstream specimen should be taken.

In **male patients**, the prepuce should be retracted and the glans washed. The patient should then start to pass urine; as he does so, many of the organisms are washed from the urinary meatus so that the first part of the specimen is liable to be heavily contaminated. This is allowed to run away. The next 50ml or so is collected into a sterile funnel dropping into a container, or into a wide-mouthed screw-cap jar. This is probably only slightly contaminated, if at all, and is used as the specimen for examination. The remainder of the urine is allowed to run away.

It is more difficult to obtain a satisfactory specimen in **female patients**. The vulva should be washed down with sterile water or saline. When the patient starts to pass urine, the first part of the specimen is discarded. About 50ml should then be collected into a wide-mouthed screw-cap jar for use as the bacteriological specimen. The remainder is discarded. If bacterial counts are required, these specimens must be sent to the laboratory immediately.

In **children**, the glans penis or vulva should be washed as in adults. Plastic bags are probably the best things to use for collecting specimens.

Sometimes an 'early morning' or '24-hour' specimen is required for examination for tubercle bacilli. The entire specimen should then be collected into a screw-cap bottle and sent to the laboratory. It is important that the bottle has not been previously used for the same purpose, as this may result in a 'false-positive' report owing to organisms from the previous specimen being left in the container.

Faeces: Faeces always contain large numbers of normal microbes apart from those which may be causing disease. It is not possible, or necessary, to obtain a sterile specimen. The patient should pass a motion into a bedpan or a wide-mouthed container; part of this, about the size of a walnut, is then removed into a screw-cap jar by means of a wooden spatula. Sometimes the whole specimen has to be sent to the laboratory, for example, when the head of a tapeworm is being looked for. In suspected cases of amoebic dysentery, the specimen must be sent to the laboratory when it is still fresh and warm. It is **essential** to warn the laboratory about this in advance.

When an open container or bedpan is sent to the laboratory, it must be properly enclosed in a plastic bag, the neck of which is firmly closed by a rubber band.

Blood cultures. These must be taken using full aseptic ritual as for a minor operation.

Specimens for virological examination are collected in much the same way as for bacteriological examination. However, it is wise to find out in advance whether the laboratory has any special requirements so far as collection, storage, and transport of the specimens is concerned.

Serological examination

The specimen required is blood obtained by venepuncture. This is a skill acquired by practice. Blood should always be collected aseptically, using a no-touch technique after the skin over the patient's vein has been swabbed with antiseptic.

The syringe must be dry and sterile. A wet syringe will cause haemolysis which will make it impossible to carry out the test. Blood should be collected into a **plain** tube, in which it is allowed to clot before the serum is removed; this is done in the laboratory. 5-10ml of blood are required; less than this may not be enough.

In most infections, antibodies begin to appear in the blood during the second week of the disease. A specimen taken in the first few days of the illness will not reveal them, unless the patient has suffered from this particular type of infection before. However, an early specimen is of value to compare with the antibody content of a specimen taken a fortnight later. If the second specimen shows a marked rise in antibody titre compared with the first, this indicates the presence of infection.

'Paired' specimens, one taken early in the illness and the second about two weeks later, should be taken whenever possible.

SELECT GLOSSARY

Abscess—A localised collection of pus formed as a result of inflammation.

Acid fast bacilli—Usually refers to tubercle bacilli, so called because, when stained, they will resist decolorisation with acid. Also refers to other members of the mycobacteria group to which the tubercle bacillus belongs.

Aerobic—Bacteria which need oxygen in order to multiply.

Anaerobic—Bacteria which are capable of multiplying in the absence of oxygen.

Agglutination—The clumping together of bacteria and other particles by specific antibodies.

Agglutinin—A type of antibody which acts on bacteria or other particles by agglutinating (clumping) them.

Allergy—An atypical reaction of the body tissues due to sensitisation by an antigen.

Antibiotic—A substance produced by a bacterium or fungus which prevents the growth of or kills other micro-organisms. Nowadays the word is sometimes used to include chemotherapeutic substances not produced by other living organisms, such as sulphonamides.

Antibody—A substance formed by the body tissues which reacts with and neutralises an antigen. Antibodies are formed as a result of stimulation by antigens. Agglutinins, antitoxins, opsonins, and precipitins are examples of different types of antibody.

Antigen—A substance which, when introduced into the body, will stimulate the production of antibodies. Most antigens are proteins; some are polysaccharides.

Antimetabolite drugs—Drugs which interfere with the metabolic processes of the body cells.

Antisepsis—The prevention of infection by application of a chemical substance which kills or prevents the growth of microbes.

Antiseptic—A chemical substance used for antisepsis.

Antitoxin—A type of antibody which specifically neutralises a toxin.

Asepsis—The prevention of microbial contamination by the exclusion or destruction of microbes.

Attenuate—To weaken the virulence of micro-organisms by growing them under artificial conditions in the laboratory.

Autoclave—An apparatus used for sterilisation by steam under pressure.

Bacillus—A rod-shaped bacterium. Also a particular group of bacteria, namely, the Anthrax group.

Capsule—A slimy mucoid cell wall which is formed by some groups of bacteria when they invade living tissues.

Carrier—A person who harbours and excretes pathogenic microbes without suffering from the disease associated with them.

Coccus—A bacterium of rounded shape—spherical, oval, or kidney-shaped.

Colony—A group of bacteria, visible to the naked eye, which has arisen by the multiplication of a single bacterium after incubation.

Commensal—Microbes which live on the surface or in the tissues of a host without doing the host any harm.

Cross-infection—Infection of a patient in hospital by microbes from another patient.

Cross-reaction—Reaction of antigen with antibody, or antibody with antigen, different from that with which reaction was intended.

Culture—(noun)—A growth of microbes.

Culture—(verb)—To grow microbes.

Disinfectant—A chemical substance used for disinfection.

Disinfection—The destruction of pathogenic microbes.

Empirical—By observation and experiment, rather than theory.

Endemic—An infection which is always found in a particular place.

Epidemic—An infection which arises in a place in which it is not usually found.

Exanthem—Febrile illness with a skin rash.

Facultative anaerobe—A bacterium which can grow under both anaerobic and aerobic conditions.

Germicide—Same as disinfectant.

Globulin—A type of protein found in the serum which includes the antibodies.

Gram negative—Staining pink by Gram's method.

Gram positive—Staining purple by Gram's method.

Gram's method—A method of biological staining by which organisms can be divided into gram positive or gram negative according to chemical substances in their cell wall.

Heaf test—A tuberculin test performed by perforating the epidermis with a spring-loaded multiple puncture 'gun'—the 'Heaf gun'.

Host—A living organism which may harbour microbes.

Hypersensitivity—A state in which a person or an animal reacts more vigorously than usual to the presence of an antigen.

IgG—Gamma globulin, the portion of the serum globulins which contains the antibodies.

Immunity—The capacity of an individual to resist infection.

Infection—The multiplication of microbes within a host.

Infectivity—The capacity of microbes to infect a host.

Inoculate—To introduce an immunising agent into a person or animal, usually by injection, also to place microbes, or material for culture, on to or into a culture medium.

Invasiveness—The capacity of microbes to invade a host.

Lyse, Lysis—The breaking up of microbial cells.

Mantoux test—A tuberculin test performed by intradermal injection of tuberculin or PPD.

Medium—Substances in which microbes are cultured in a laboratory.

Micron—1/1000 of a millimetre.

Motile—Capable of independent movement.

Opsonin—A type of antibody which makes microbes more liable to ingestion by leucocytes.

Pathogenic—Disease producing.

Phage type—A sub-division of a particular group of microbes, such as staphylococci, based on the action of bacteriophages.

Phagocytosis—The ingestion, or adsorption, of microbes by cells such as leucocytes.

PPD—'Purified protein derivative'—an extract of tubercle bacilli used in tuberculin tests.

Precipitin—A type of antibody which reacts with an antigen in solution, producing a precipitate which is a mixture of the antigen and the antibody.

Prophylaxis—Prevention.

Pure culture—A culture of a single type of microbe.

Pyogenic—A type of infection associated with the production of pus.

Rickettsia—A type of microbe intermediate in size and other properties between bacteria and viruses.

Schick test—A skin test for susceptibility to diphtheria. A positive result denotes susceptibility, a negative result denotes immunity.

Sporadic—Occasional.

Spore—The resulting phase of certain types of bacteria, e.g., the Bacillus (anthrax) group and the Clostridia. Spores are very resistant to heat, cold, drying, and the action of chemical disinfectants. They can remain viable (alive) for very long periods in a state of 'suspended animation'.

Sterilisation—Destruction of all living microbes.

Sub-clinical infection—Infection of which the patient is unaware, and which does not produce symptoms or signs.

Toxigenicity—Capacity to produce toxins.

Toxin—A substance produced by microbes which has a damaging effect on the tissues of a susceptible animal.

Tuberculin—An extract of tubercle bacilli used in tuberculin tests.

Tuberculin test—A test for allergy to tubercle bacilli. A positive result denotes resistance to tuberculosis as well as allergy.

Vaccinate—To immunise.

Vaccine—A substance used for immunisation.

Virulence—The capacity of the microbe to cause disease.

Virus—The smallest group of micro-organisms, which cannot reproduce outside the living cells of a host. Viruses range in size from that of the smallest bacteria down to that of large protein molecules.

INDEX